為之法令終而不滅久而不絕易用難忘為
之經紀異其章別其表裏為之終始令各有
衝太衝二陰中之至陰腎也其原出於太白
太白二陰中之太陰脾也其原出於太谿太
谿二膏之原出於鳩尾鳩尾一盲之原出於
脖胦脖胦一凡此十二原者主治五藏六府
之有疾者也脹取三陽飧泄取三陰今夫五
藏之有疾也譬猶刺也猶污也猶結也猶閉
也刺雖久猶可拔也污雖久猶可雪也結雖
久猶可解也閉雖久猶可決也或言久疾之
不可取者非其說也夫善用鍼者取其疾也
猶拔刺也猶雪污也猶解結也猶決閉也疾
雖久猶可畢也言不可治者未得其術也刺
諸熱者如以手探湯刺寒清者如人不欲行
陰有陽疾者取之下陵三里正往無殆氣下
乃止不下復始也疾高而內者取之陰之陵
泉疾高而外者取之陽之陵泉也

**Extracts from the 12-volume *Miraculous Pivot*, concerned mainly with acupuncture.
In particular, these pages describe practitioners of the ancient therapy as using nine different
needles to administer treatment. Nine needles practice fell into disuse, and was only revived recently.**

萬物之終始也死生之本也逆之則災害生從之則苛疾不起是謂得道道者聖人行之愚者佩之從陰陽則生逆之則死從之則治逆之則亂反順為逆是謂內格是故聖人不治已病治未病不治已亂治未亂此之謂也夫病已成而後藥之亂已成而後治之譬猶渴而穿井鬬而鑄兵不亦晚乎

○生氣通天論篇第三

黃帝曰夫自古通天者生之本本於陰陽天地之間六合之內其氣九州九竅五藏十二

黃帝素問靈樞經卷之一

○九鍼十二原第一 法天

黃帝問於歧伯曰余子萬民養百姓而收其租稅余哀其不給而屬有疾病余欲勿使被

Unbelievable Cures & Medicines From China

China Features

NEW WORLD PRESS, BEIJING

First Edition 1997
Copyright © 1997 by CHINA FEATURES
P.O. Box 522, Beijing 100803, China

In accordance with the Copyright Law of
the People's Republic of China, 1991

All rights reserved. No part of this work may be reproduced
in any form by any means without the written
permission of the copyright owner.

ISBN 7-80005-322-9

First Published by
NEW WORLD PRESS
24 Baiwanzhuang Road, Beijing 100037, China

Distributed by
CHINA INTERNATIONAL BOOK TRADING CORPORATION
35 Chegongzhuang Xilu, Beijing 100044, China
P.O. Box 399, Beijing, China

Contents

Preface
Introduction: TCMs Balanced Approach to Health
1. A Medicine to Move Mountains ... 1
2. Fighting Poison with Poison ... 5
3. A Herbal Injection to Cure Epilepsy ... 14
4. Forgotten Points of Acupuncture ... 20
5. Taking the Pain out of Conquering the Big C ... 25
6. A Deadly Weed: Medicine in Medical Hands ... 33
7. The Point of Heat ... 38
8. Putting Ants to Work on Arthritis ... 44
9. Removing Sources of Pain with the Blade-Tipped Needle ... 49
10. A Pharmacy in a Tiny Bottle ... 61
11. Threads Soaked in Mystery ... 68
12. Making Life Liveable with AIDS ... 74
13. Easing Cold Turkey Traumas ... 80
14. A Hair Raiser for Wig Wearers ... 87
15. South China's Pharmaceutical Institution ... 93
16. A Herbal Swipe at Malaria ... 99
17. Scalp Acupuncture: Therapy Close to the Site of Strokes ... 105
18. Attacking the Parasitic Culprit of Acne ... 111
19. Remedies from Forest and Family ... 116
20. A Break from Traditional Patience ... 121
21. For the Health of Newborn Babies ... 126
22. Detecting Signals of Distress from Tumors ... 133
23. Teaming up with Nature to Beautify ... 139
24. Breathing Life Back into the Paralysed ... 145
25. The World of the Medicine King ... 152
26. Evidencing the Evolution of Chinese Medicine ... 157
Appendix (Writers & Contact Information)
Postscript: Behind the Book

Preface

To a large extent, Western medicine has become world medicine. With globalization, the majority of the world's sick and diseased have come to rely on chemically-synthesized drugs to effect cures. Yet despite the advancement of Western medical science, drugs sometimes fail to work, and many of them induce side effects.

Yet the majority of China's 1.2 billion population still use *Zhongyi*, or traditional Chinese medicine (TCM), for solutions to health problems. With a 5,000-year-long history, the practice offers natural, safe but nonetheless effective therapies and cures for many diseases. On this basis — unparalleled history and sheer number of benefactors — TCM can claim to be *Eastern* medicine.

TCM differs in a fundamental way from Western medicine, but there is an overlap, where East meets West. Many contemporary TCM practitioners have actually undergone training in Western medicine. And one area where the two schools are similar is in their quests for progress. TCM is, by definition, traditional, but that in no way prevents it from evolving.

Some of the latest TCM breakthroughs are introduced in this book UNBELIEVABLE CURES & MEDICINES FROM CHINA.

The entirely new practice of *acupotomy*, for example, uses an instrument which is part acupuncture needle, part surgical scalpel. Practitioners across China are using the needle-scalpel daily to treat at least 10,000 patients suffering from musculoskeletal complaints. Variations on standard acupuncture are also a prominent revival-cum-development: needles of various shape and size which fell into disuse are once again being used in improved forms, and now, administered with heat or magnetism, are proving their worth in the teatment of hosts of traumatic injuries and internal maladies. Meanwhile, ingredients which may seem quite strange to foreigners — ants, snake venom and the root sap of toxic plants — form active components in medicines which cure arthritis, cerebrovascular diseases and epilepsy.

However, ingredients are not the only part of TCM to baffle foreigners. The Chinese system is fundamentally different from Western medicine in its approach: TCM theory hinges on the concept of wholism, stressing the overall, delicate harmony and coordination among different parts of the human body, and the careful readjustment and maintenance of this natural balance. For this reason, an introductory chapter is included to define and explain the principle theories behind TCM.

Ignorance notwithstanding, there are other reasons why much of the world should have remained mystified by TCM: secrecy has long surrounded the preparation of many traditional Chinese medicines, imperial courts of past dynasties shunned their empires' participation in foreign trade, political upheavals induced further isolation and most of all, the language barrier has always hindered the free and easy exchange of information.

It is through a desire to promote a better understanding of TCM that this book has been published.

Of course, what is presented here is but a page from a vast library. Yet the book provides an opportunity for foreigners to glean a better understanding of some TCM treatments being used and practiced in the mid-1990s. And for the convenience of those in the medical profession, medical students, patients and their relatives interested in following up on particular treatments, contact information has been listed in an appendix.

Written by journalists with no medical training themselves, the book is easy reading despite its many medical concepts, conditions and treatments. Writers and editors hope it serves to evidence TCM's suitability as an effective alternative to Western medicine for certain diseases, and in the process help people recover from illnesses and live healthier lives.

The Editors,
June, 1997

Introduction

TCMs BALANCED APPROACH TO HEALTH

It is difficult for non-Chinese to comprehend traditional Chinese medicine (TCM) as the practice is entirely different from their native approaches.

The purpose of this introductory chapter is to give readers a basic understanding of TCM theories before they explore the core chapters dealing with prominent developments within the practice.

Western medicine is a precise science. The minds of its doctors have, from the outset of their training, been instructed to deal with the proven and fixed whether they be concepts, laws or quantities.

Whereas Western doctors tend to address a patient's problem in a relatively isolated way by treating the infected or injured part directly, the TCM practitioner takes a broad, macroscopic view and treats the body as a whole.

Traditional Chinese medicine is much more than a science. It is a history, an art, a culture and a belief. But the most prominent component of TCM is the cosmic element. The Chinese have, for 5,000 years, regarded the human body as a microcosm of universal order. This vision has as its central tenet an analogy of the body with mother nature, and was first formulated by the sage Lao Zi in the 6th century BC. His ideas bore fluorescence in Daoism, China's only indigenous religion and philosophy, if not traditional way of life.

Qi: Vital Energy

The major premise of TCM is that all living things, including people, have a life force within them. This vital biological energy, which is invisible, is known as *qi* to the Chinese. It is innate from the moment of our conception, after which it is generated or degenerated according to external factors, most importantly the environment (weather), particularly the air which we breathe, and internally as the nourishment we make available by our digestion of food.

TCM practitioners believe that a person's health suffers when vital energy is at a low ebb. Consequently, as an important part of diagnostic procedure, TCM practitioners try to ascertain their patient's psychological outlook, general life style and routine for pointers as to what has become imbalanced. Only as a last resort is medicine prescribed. Chinese doctors are happier if they can solve their patient's problems with dietary, breathing exercise or hygienic advice.

Herbal medicines can revitalize *qi,* the body's vital energy. Certain plants and animal ingredients have natural affinities with internal organs, hence a skillful TCM practitioner can prescribe a medicine which will act curatively, often indirectly, on the problem area while inflicting no harm on the body's natural and sensitive equilibrium. Speed of function may be slower, but safer, than chemically-synthesized Western medicines, which often cause side effects.

Yin-Yang

Daoism further influenced the evolution of traditional Chinese medicine with its abstract theory of *yin-yang* forces which emerged circa 6th century BC.

Yin is a negative, calm force. It is characterized by the female gender and symbolized by water. *Yang* is the opposite force, positive and active in nature. It is characterized by the male gender and is symbolized by fire. The interaction of negative-positive, of female-male, water-fire and so on is believed to produce all change and motion in the cosmic sphere.

From reading the properties of *yin* and *yang*, one might consider *yang*, as male and active, to be superior to *yin*, which is female and passive. However, Daoists have, from time immemorial, regarded *yin* as the superior of the two forces: the word always precedes *yang* when spoken and written. While fire is powerful and capable of flaring up quickly, it can be doused by water. Moreover, given eons of time, water can erode a mountain.

Regardless of which force is superior, the body functions at its best when the two forces are balanced in relative terms. Imbalances tend to occur from season to season, especially when the weather changes, or when a person travels from one environment to another. Although the body can redress *yin-yang* imbalances within certain limits, *yin* and *yang* foods can help effect speedier readjustments.

The Chinese are totally aware of this: their eating habits are governed by *yin-yang* considerations, and in this respect all parents imbue dietary-medical advice on their children from an early age. Any Westerner invited to a Chinese banquet will learn that a particular food's nutritional value is often discussed and may even be the reason for its appearance on the table. This also explains why such an array of different foods appear at one meal.

Only when self-administered attempts to redress the imbalance of *yin-yang* are unsuccessful is medicine prescribed. When diagnosing, the practitioner factors in weather, seasonal and geographical considerations, and tries to differentiate between the *yin* and *yang* nature of the disease.

Five Elements (*Wu Xing*)

All matter on the planet has a dominant character which bears resemblance to the properties of one of the five elements: Metal (*jin*), Wood (*mu*), Water (*shui*), Fire (*huo*) and Earth (*tu*). Together with the interaction of *yin-yang*, interplay among the five elements is the prime mover to explain all activities in nature. According to China's earliest extant medical work, *The Yellow Emperor's Internal Classic*: "Metal, Wood, Water, Fire and Earth encompass all natural phenomena. This symbolism also applies to man." In other words, all parts of the human body have affinities in nature with a particular element.

The Chinese liken organs in the human body to the five elements to symbolize their cyclic inter-relationship, inter-dependence and generation-subjugation relationships. It should be stressed that this is a symbolic recognition — an analogy. Particularly, the organ-element analogies are lung(s)-Metal; liver-Wood; kidney(s)-Water; heart-Fire; and spleen-Earth.

This analogy broadens out to encompass all components of the body, since each and every part of the anatomy is controlled by a particular vital organ. Specifically, the heart controls blood circulation; lungs control the skin; liver, the tendons; spleen, the muscles; and kidneys, the bones.

In practice, that is why, for example, a TCM practitioner treats a skin problem with medication for its corresponding vital organ — the lungs — which controls the supply of vital energy to the skin. A Western doctor, in contrast, is likely to treat the skin directly, perhaps by prescribing an ointment which can be applied externally to the skin.

Regarding cyclic-relationships among the organs and one-to-one relationships between them, two complete cycles and numerous one-to-one relationships are recognized. The positive cycle is initiated by Wood, which burns to make Fire, leaving a pile of ashes to generate Earth. Earth generates Metal which can be mined from the ground. Metal melts when heated, and flows like Water. The liquid promotes the growth of plants and thus generates Wood.

The negative cycle is also initiated by Wood (plants) which subjugates Earth by breaking up the soil and extracting its nutrients. Earth subjugates Water by containing it and soiling its purity. Water subjugates Fire by extinguishing it. Fire subjugates Metal by melting it and Metal subjugates Wood by cutting it.

One-to-one relationships are described either being mother-son or victor-vanquished in character. An example of the former would be Fire, which is mother to son Earth (it burns to make ashes which forms Earth). But Fire is also son to mother Wood — without Wood there can be no Fire.

The significance of all these analogies is their link with the vital organs and their inter-relationships. The analogy allows the practitioner to understand how one organ has relative influences on others.

The Vital Organs (*Zang-Fu* Organs)

The vital organs consist of two groups: the five solid organs (*wu zang*), and the six hollow organs (*liu fu*).

The five solid organs are the heart, lungs, liver, kidneys and spleen. The six hollow organs are the small intestine, large intestine, gall bladder, urinary bladder, stomach and the *san jiao*. This latter member, which translates as "triple warmer", is not really an organ, and therefore doesn't exist in Western medicine. It is divided into the upper, middle and lower *jiao*. The upper *jiao* houses the heart and lung; the middle houses the spleen and stomach, while the lower houses the liver, kidneys, urinary bladder, small and large intestines. The function of the *san jiao* (upper, middle and lower) represents the summation of those grouped vital *zang-fu* organs. They are also the passageways of *qi* and body fluids.

Balance, as one must fully realize, is absolutely essential to order, and health. Since five does not balance six, an extra solid organ is added to the *wu zang* grouping. It is the pericardium which envelops the heart.

The solid organs are *yin* in character while the hollow ones are *yang*. Each pairing of solid-hollow organs resembles one of the five elements in nature.

Meridian System (*Jingluo*)

Any illness is said to reflect the malfunction of one of the coupled pairs of organs, which of course initiates a negative, knock-on effect on the others.

The organs are connected physically, both Chinese and Western medicine agree, by circulatory, lymphatic and nervous connections which transport blood, other body fluids and messages respectively.

But TCM practitioners believe in the existence of hosts of other connections, *jingluo*, or channels and collaterals, a dendritic system of conduits for the circulation of blood and *qi*, vital energy, throughout the body. The channels are the main conduits, deeply situated. The collaterals form a subsidiary network interconnecting the channels. Together they function to interlink the solid and hollow organs, the muscles, tendons, bones, and sensory organs, thus making the body an organic whole.

Acupuncturists can select points on the body surface in the vicinity of appropriate channels and collaterals at which to insert their needles. Rotation of the needle then effects stimulation which is transmitted along the channels and collaterals to the vital organ which hosts the root cause of the complaint.

This explains why, for example, a practitioner addressing a problem in the patient's eye actually puts needles in the patient's ear auricle. This "remote" attention to disease is a peculiarity of TCM, while a Western doctor would almost certainly treat the eye directly.

Moreover, the ear is regarded as a miniature fetus (upside down), and acupuncture in the ear auricle can therefore have a therapeutic effect on every single part of the body.

It must be fully understood that since every part of the body is linked to a particular vital organ via the meridian system of channels and collaterals (*jingluo*), any ailment can be tackled by focusing treatment on the controlling vital organ.

Summary

Qi, *yin-yang*, the five elements (*wu xing*), *zang-fu* organs and *jingluo* are terms, concepts and theories totally alien in Western medicine, yet form the basis for understanding traditional Chinese medicine in its native place. In China and neighboring countries influenced by Chinese culture, including Japan, Korea and southeast Asian nations, these terms and the theories behind them are common knowledge.

Qi is vital energy present to greater or lesser degrees in all living things. It circulates along *jingluo*, a meridian system, around the body. Within the body, the forces of *yin-yang* are at play, relative balance of which ensures good health. All parts of the anatomy are likened to the five elements by way of corresponding vital organs. The Chinese recognize a group of 12 organs as being vital: these are subdivided into the solid and hollow groups which in turn control each and every part of the anatomy, either directly or indirectly via the meridian system.

Western medicine does not accept theories which cannot be measured. It is a science that concerns itself with the location and structure of organs and biochemical analysis of tissues. Its doctors focus on problems in isolation during diagnoses and treatment.

In contrast, TCM practitioners treat the body as an inseparable whole which is attune with nature. Illnesses, mental or physical, are regarded as clear indications of the body's *yin-yang* imbalances. Treatment may involve improving the diet or prescribing herbal medicines, either *yin* or *yang* in nature, to readjust the body's *yin-yang* balance to a state of healthy equilibrium.

CHAPTER 1

A MEDICINE TO MOVE MOUNTAINS

Gallstones, afflicting one in ten adults, give excruciating abdominal pain. Pai Shi San is a no pain, no gain medicine, but highly effective. Chinese traditional medicine practitioner, Wang Changgen, has used his herbal preparation to force thousands of stones down bile ducts in a process which he says is akin to childbirth.

Cai Enyou, aged 18, was as frail as a straw: at 1.7 meters, he weighed only 40 kilograms. He was often bent double in pain. The cause of his mal-health: gallstones.

Cai's parents, natives of Wenling County in East China's Zhejiang Province, sought a cure for their son in five hospitals, spending a small fortune in the process. But the pain continued to afflict the boy.

Then, in 1990, the family heard of a "miracle" doctor and visited his small clinic situated in the center of Hangzhou, the provincial capital of Zhejiang. The boy was prescribed 27 packages of herbal medicine and, within 25 days of taking it, he passed 3 gallstones in his stools. Two of the stones combined measured 9.3 x 4.2cm. Since ridding himself of the stones he has enjoyed good health.

Cai Enyou is one of hundreds of thousands of gallstone sufferers who owe their new lives to Dr. Wang Changgen, 55, a self-taught doctor practicing traditional Chinese medicine.

Dr. Wang and his 49-year-old wife, Lang Jingfen, operate a private clinic offering specialized treatment to gallstone sufferers at 317, Zhongshan Road: a stone's throw from Hangzhou's scenic West Lake.

There is often standing room only in the clinic for waiting patients. Jars containing gallstones from cured patients are displayed on Dr. Wang's desk and cabinets. One room, filled with sacks of herbs, serves as the pharmacy.

Akin to Childbirth

"My idea is simple," Dr. Wang says with a strong local accent. "I use a combination of herbs that essentially do two things: enlarge the bile duct and increase the secretion of bile."

He explains that an enlarged bile duct allows stones to pass down to the intestines, and the increased quantity of bile in the gallbladder creates a pressure on the stones, to push them out, as well as lubricating the duct to ease the stones' passage — the process of gallstone removal is similar to childbirth. However, this raises a question: "Will stones, on their way out, injure the bile duct?"

"No," the doctor says. "Gallstones are soft while inside the body, only hardening when exposed to air. My method of treatment has never caused any internal bleeding."

Prior Inducement of Pain

Dr. Wang says his medicine works best when the patient feels pain. With such patients, the rate of successful gallstone removal reaches 98 percent, according to an investigation on patients treated by Wang from 1990-91.

"When the patient feels pain, the gallstones are active and are thus pushed out more easily by bile pressure," he says. This explains the radical departure from conventional wisdom in Dr. Wang's treatment: the inducement of pain.

"I advise my patients to eat high-protein and high-fat foods, or simply get tired, to induce pain. Then they should take the medicine when the pain starts, and continue taking doses until the gallstones come out."

"Pain indicates that the stones are on their way out. But such pain is mild, compared with how the patient felt when the gallstones were 'active' prior to treatment," he says.

Wang's treatment is also effective for getting rid of liver stones. He concedes that 30 percent of patients who fail to induce pain do not pass gallstones after taking his medicine.

"This is due to an absence of stones in some patients as well as to the occasional failure of the medicine in certain cases, but the medicine removes symptoms all the same," he says. He uses exceptionally large doses. One prescription often amounts to 20-30 packages. Patients take the medicine at home, thus avoiding hospitalization. Gallstones are removed within 2-3 days of taking the medicine in the quickest cases, and within two months in the slowest, he claims.

Dr. Wang has so far treated approximately 400,000 patients, including a considerable number from overseas. His reputation initially spread mainly by word of mouth. In the last five years, press and media coverage at home and abroad have further spread news about his successful treatment.

A Concentrate is Born

Wang's medicine consists of more than 10 ordinary herbs and a powder he calls *Pai Shi San*, or Stone Removal Promoter. The crucial part of his prescription is this *Pai Shi San*, which is made up of three herbs and prepared by the Wangs at home.

Understandably, for commercial reasons, the making of *Pai Shi San* is a secret. But Dr. Wang does not shun technological processes in the medicine's manufacture. Beginning in 1991, in cooperation with the Shantou No. 2 Pharmaceutical Factory, he has been producing a capsuled concentrate of his medicine. It has the same efficacy as decocted or self-simmered herbs prescribed by the doctor. He calls the concentrate *Dan Tong Wang*.

Since its factory manufacture, the concentrate has won numerous awards at home and abroad. For example, at the Chinese Science & Technology Achievements Exhibition held in Jakarta, Indonesia, in January 1992, *Dan Tong Wang* concentrate won the only gold medal among 1,300 exhibits. During the exhibition, Dr. Wang treated with success a VIP patient: President Suharto's brother-in-law. News of the cure spread fast and the 6,000 capsules supply of *Dan Tong Wang* in Indonesia was sold out in no time.

Ambassador of Cross-Straits Exchanges

Soon after his return from Indonesia, Dr. Wang Changgen visited Taiwan as "an outstanding mainland personage." On March 20, 1992, Chen Li-fu, once Chiang Kai-shek's right hand man, received Dr. Wang in Taipei. The 93-year-old Chen expressed his appreciation for his guest's unique treatment and wrote a calligraphic inscription for him, which reads: "Developing traditional Chinese medicine to ease pain for patients the world over."

In Taichung, in cooperation with a local doctor, Jiang Hechun, Dr. Wang set up a clinic named after himself. Wang supplies the clinic with herbs and *Dan Tong Wang* concentrate. The clinic has treated thousands of patients in the last few years.

Dr. Wang has set up other clinics in a host of major Chinese cities in cooperation with local hospitals. These cities include Beijing, Tianjin, Wuhan, Taiyuan and Luoyang. Overseas, he has appointed sales agents for his *Dan Tong Wang* concentrate in Singapore, Malaysia and Japan.

From Cotton Mill Heir to Self-Made Doctor

Though the son of a cotton mill owner, young Wang was not interested in textiles but in traditional medicine. Through self-study of books and plants, he familiarized himself at an early age with medicinal herbs and became a recognized authority in the field.

His search for a successful gallstone treatment began at a Hangzhou community hospital, where, as a doctor specializing in the treatment of the digestive system, he found that problems of the gallbladder were often wrongly attributed to the stomach. "Since one in every 10 people suffer from gallstones, I decided to concentrate on their removal," he says.

He spent ten years trying to find a cure. "I've benefited immensely from works by ancient herbalists and doctors," he says.

Despite success and a busy schedule treating patients, Dr. Wang continues to do much research work.

"I need to further improve my dispensing as well as look for cures for other related diseases," he says.

CHAPTER 2

FIGHTING POISON WITH POISON

To be bitten by a Pallas pit viper, one of Asia's most poisonous snakes, would mean death by unstoppable bleeding. Realizing that the hemorrhaging component of snake bite could be useful in certain medical situations, Hao Wenxue set out to turn a bad thing into a good thing. And after many years in the lab and field observing and catching the deadly reptiles, he finally formulated his venom-based anti-thrombus medicine to remove clots.

If blood forms a clot in the vessels of the human brain, the patient faces one of three fates: instant death, paralysis, or paralysis of one side of the body.

Cerebrovascular diseases have always been a serious threat to the middle-aged and elderly. In recent years in China, for example, cerebrovascular diseases have struck down about 2.4 million people annually, making them more of a killer than cancer, according to figures from the China National Cerebrovascular Diseases Prevention and Treatment Office.

No breakthroughs have so far been made in the search for a cure for such diseases. But a Chinese professor has invented an unconventional method of dealing with them. He uses an injection refined from snake venom.

Hao Wenxue, 70, a professor with China Medical University in Shenyang, capital of Liaoning Province, has devoted 30 years to snake venom research. The latest result of his work is an injection called Svate-3 (*Ahalysantinfarctasum*), which has been used to treat more than 100,000 cerebrovascular cases in 300 hospitals across China. It has proved most effective when treating cerebral thrombosis, or blood clotting in the brain's blood vessels, a condition commonly known as a stroke.

The injection has the functions of preventing coagulation, dissolving clots, lowering blood fat levels, dilating blood vessels and improving microcirculation. More importantly, the injection contains a nerve growth factor (NGF) that reinforces the functions of the nerve cell.

Snake Venom

In spite of its toxicity, venom from poisonous snakes has, for a long time, been valued by practitioners of traditional Chinese medicine as an effective compound for treating some difficult and complicated diseases. "To fight poison with poison," the theory goes.

Venom is spurted from a snake's fangs when the animal faces threat or preys on a predator. It is the reptile's digestion fluid, attack and self-defense weapon.

Snake venom contains a number of deadly toxins. They include a neurotoxin which attacks the central nervous system to cause paralysis and suffocation to death, and a hemotoxin that causes the bleeding of internal organs and circulation failure, which often results in death. In addition, snake venom contains a cardiotoxin that causes palpitation and a musculartoxin which freezes muscle movement.

However, snake venom also contains non-toxic or low-toxicity enzymes and proteins. The most important is an enzyme which has the property of dissolving blood clots in vessels. It is called the anti-thrombus enzyme.

The key to using snake venom for the treatment of diseases rests with the biochemist's ability to successfully separate the beneficial compounds from the harmful ones.

Use of the snake venom for medical purposes dates back to ancient times in China. Li Shizhen (1518-93), a well-known medical scientist of the Ming Dynasty (1368-1644), wrote in his *Compendium of Materia Medica* regarded as the Bible of Chinese traditional pharmacy: "The *Pallas* pit viper can relieve paralysis of one half of the body (hemiplegia)." In traditional Chinese medicine, all parts of the snake are regarded as having medical values.

Up to now, about 2,200 species of snakes have been found worldwide, of which 600 are poisonous. There are 160 species in China, and 10 of them are poisonous.

The *Pallas* pit viper, a very poisonous species, is distributed across most of China except Tibet, Guangdong and Guangxi.

According to a report published in 1963 on 10 patients in Malaysia who were bitten by the viper, the patients' unstoppable bleeding was due to a thrombinoid, an enzyme contained in the pit viper's venom. It prevented their blood from coagulating. In other words, the report implied that the snake venom could do something desirable: dissolve blood clots. The finding spurred researchers in the field to develop a medicine for cerebrovascular diseases from snake venom.

Work in this area, however, has been difficult, obviously because of the dangers involved in capturing snakes and removing venom from their fangs.

When he was a child, Hao Wenxue dreamed of building roads and bridges for the local community, an ambition he inherited from his great grandfather. Although he built no roads or bridges after growing up and becoming a doctor, his ambition of doing something for the public good stayed with him. And so he took it upon himself to extract medicine from snake venom, a task that he knew was going to be difficult.

After graduation from the China Medical University in Shenyang in the 1950s, Hao became a chest surgeon. A frequent witness to pains suffered by those undergoing surgery, he dreamed that one day he might develop a medicine that could dispense with the need for surgery on cancer patients.

One day in May 1965, Hao received a patient and, after careful diagnosis, he found that the man was suffering advanced stage cancer of the esophagus. He thought the patient would not live for another month. But, two months later, the patient returned, very much alive. He told Hao that he had been drinking "snake soup" prescribed by a snake seller named Fan Hansheng. The doctor immediately paid a visit to Fan to find out more.

Ever since then, Prof. Hao has been engrossed in the study of snakes. Yet he has always, and still does, harbor an innate fear of the dangerous reptiles. To do his work, he bought snakes and even raised them at home. He became a student of Qin Yaoting, a professor of biology at Liaoning University, in his quest to gain as much knowledge as possible about serpents. And it was in August 1965 that Hao Wenxue finally decided to put down his scalpel and instead devote himself fully to developing an anti-cancer medicine from snake venom.

Cerebral Thrombosis

When developing the first generation of the snake venom injection (Svate-1), Hao Wenxue was actually searching for a cancer cure.

Jiang Kaiqi was suffering from stomach cancer. Svate-1 did very little to cure it, but it greatly alleviated the swelling of his lower leg. That had resulted from poor blood flow, which in turn had been caused by poor treatment of Jiang's leg when it was broken in his youth. By default, it dawned on Prof. Hao that Svate-1 possessed the property of dissolving blood clots (or acting as an anti-thrombus). Immediately, he thought of Svate-1's possible curative effect on cerebral thrombosis.

The second generation of the snake venom injection (Svate-2) developed by Prof. Hao passed a state assessment in 1985. Its sole production right was sold to the Shenyang No.1 Pharmaceutical Factory for 6 million yuan (US$750,000).

Nonetheless, Svate-2 was not completely free of the neurotoxins and hemotoxins found in snake venom. Clinical observations proved that high-dose treatment, due to these impurities, would cause toxic reactions such as double vision and bleeding.

All medicines have an appropriate dosage standard. If the dose is too low, the medicine will be ineffective; if too high, it will be harmful, inducing serious side effects.

To ascertain the optimum dosage, Hao Wenxue self-injected snake venom on five occasions, so as to personally experience his body's reactions to the compounds. A couple of times he made himself dreadfully ill. Meanwhile, his work often took him out of the lab, away from home, and into the field on a hunt for snakes. He visited Snake Island off Dalian in the Bohai Sea more than 100 times as a member of an investigation team. He recalls: "At first, I stayed on the island for six months. To understand the habits and characteristics of snakes at night, I would observe one creature for hours. I kept up these studies for eight years."

In 1985, Hao invested 3 million yuan of his own money in building a special hospital, the Dalian Senile Diseases Prevention, Treatment and Research Center. Located on the coast with 50 beds, the hospital serves as his clinical and research base. In this idyllic, picturesque setting overlooking the sea, Hao Wenxue developed the third generation of his snake venom injection (Svate-3). It took him five years.

Svate-3 passed an assessment conducted by the Ministry of Public Health in December 1991. Experts involved in the assessment evaluated the medicine as the best of its kind in China and deemed Hao's research as having reached an international level.

Prof. Chen Yuancong of the Shanghai Biochemical Research Institute under the Chinese Academy of Sciences played a pivotal role in Hao's development of Svate-3. It was Chen who helped Hao successfully develop the technique to separate neurotoxin and hemotoxin from snake venom. Patients can now be injected with 12 doses of Svate-3 in one single treatment through a neck artery.

Prof. Chen has devoted himself to the study of protein chemistry for 40 years. He says: "I've produced many research results, but only by cooperating with Prof. Hao Wenxue have I tasted the pleasure of doing good for mankind."

Effective

The Yangtze River Basin is a prime habitat for *Pallas* pit vipers. Jiangxi, Jiangsu and Zhejiang provinces are reputed to export about a million pit vipers a year to Japan, where snake wines are popular. They are believed to generally fortify the body, in particular inducing aphrodisiacal effects.

Venom collected in those provinces, called *Agkistrodon Hyals Pallas*, is the major source of Hao's medicine. Hao uses six components of the venom as ingredients of his Svate-3. They are separated by a complex process.

Animal (dog) experiments and 10,000 cases of clinical application have proved that Svate-3 is effective in treating cerebral thrombosis in all its different stages. In addition, it is effective in treating diabetes. High dose and local perfusion methods are particularly effective. Toxicological tests have shown that Svate-3, free of neurotoxin and hemotoxin, is safe and reliable. It does no harm to the liver nor kidneys.

Deng Guoxiang, 67, was sent to the Dalian Senile Diseases Center in March 1991 suffering from acute cerebral thrombosis and diabetes. When carried to the emergency room on a stretcher, he could hardly

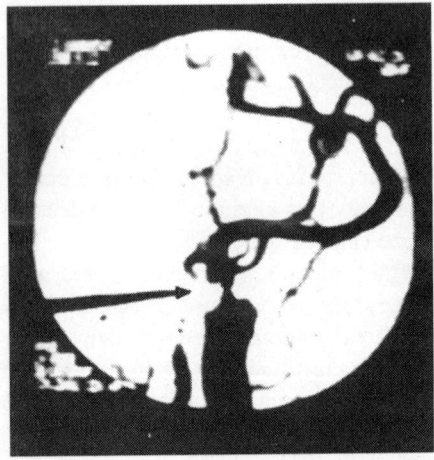

DSA (Digital Subtraction Angiograthy), before treatment.

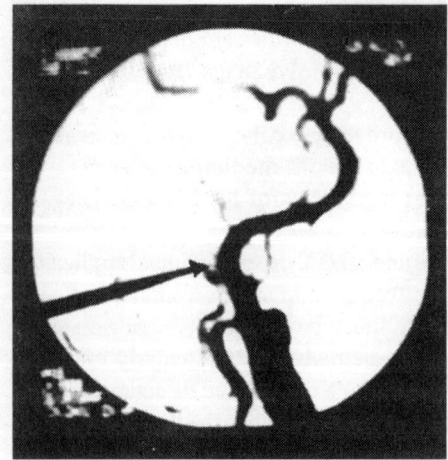

DSA (Digital Subtraction Angiograthy), after treatment.

speak, swallow or move. After two-days' treatment, 20 doses a day, he could speak clearly, stand up and walk freely for 7-10 meters.

Retired shoemaker Feng Kelin, 74, was paralyzed due to thrombosis of the middle cerebral artery. After 50 days' treatment, 8 doses per day, he could soon walk 100 meters by himself.

In November 1991, a Japanese patient went to Hao's hospital. He had been diagnosed in Japan as suffering from coronary thrombosis and told that neither an operation nor medicine could help him. But after undergoing a 45-day treatment program on Svate-3 in Dalian, the thrombus in his heart was gone.

During the China Scientific and Technological Achievements Exhibition held in Indonesia in January 1992, Hao Wenxue visited a 69-year-old local woman whose right side was paralyzed. After three doses of Svate-3, introduced by intravenous drip for 10 minutes, she could move her right hand; three days later, she could lift her hand up to her head; five days later she could get up and walk.

Associate Professor Li Xuejuan, 54, director of the ward in Hao's hospital, who has treated 1,000 patients, says: "Svate-3 is more effective than *Batroxobin* imported from Japan, as well as *Urokinase* and *Dextrani*, also commonly prescribed. The effect of *Urokinase*, for example, can only last four hours, whereas Svate-3 remains effective for 8-12 hours."

Intravenous drip and rest have long been the combined standard treatment for cerebral thrombosis patients. Since 1989, Hao Wenxue has cooperated with Jinzhou Central Hospital in using the internationally advanced Digital Subtraction Angiography (DSA) method that delivers Svate-3 right to the thrombotic focus through a catheter (a tubular device through which a liquid can be directed). The advantage of the method is that it allows the doctor to visually monitor the changes brought about by the medicine in the affected blood vessels for a period of two hours.

Dream

According to Dr. Zhang Jinxiang of the hospital, 50 cases of DSA clinical application within two years evidence Svate-3's effectiveness. Patient Yang Jingjiang, for example, could slowly raise her paralyzed arm after treatment. Yang said excitedly: "This medicine really works."

Hao Wenxue realized that it was necessary to commercialize his research findings and enable him to use whatever profit he made for funding further research into the medical uses of snake venom.

In 1990, he invested 6 million yuan (US$800,000) in the joint establishment of the Dalian Svate Pharmaceutical Co. with a Hong Kong company. Later, he founded the Hao Snake Venom Development Corporation Group. Both the company and group produce Svate-brand venom products, including Svate-3, NGF (nerve growth factor) and *Shuganmei*, a medicine especially effective for treating Hepatitis B. The brand name, Svate, is an acronym for Snake Venom Anti-Thrombosis Enzyme.

As a scholar-entrepreneur, Hao Wenxue aims to produce first-class products and step into the international market, especially those in Southeast Asia, Europe and America.

Hao's factory, located in the outskirts of Dalian, currently produces 12 million doses of Svate-3 per year, with an output value of 20 million yuan (US$2.5 million). Under his auspices, a national snake venom-related research, production and application network has taken shape.

News of the snake venom-based medicine has motivated patients to travel to Dalian to see Hao Wenxue from Japan, Indonesia, the Republic of Korea, the Philippines, Hong Kong and Taiwan. Almost all of them have enjoyed recoveries to varying degrees after being treated with Svate products.

Zhou Deming and his son, both from Taiwan, went to Dalian in spring 1996. Suffering from heart disease, the father often feels numbness in the hands. The son has congenital cerebellum atrophy and diabetes. The 59-year-old father said: "We were recommended to come to Dalian. We have confidence in Hao Wenxue's snake venom medicine."

A South Korean patient wrote to Hao Wenxue to say that it was Svate-3 that gave him strength to live on.

According to Gu Binxiang, an associate professor of the Senile Diseases Prevention Center, overseas patients should contact the center first to arrange a program of treatment before coming to China. Doctors and nurses at the center can speak a little English, therefore daily dialogues on treatment will not pose a problem.

Hao Wenxue travels around the country, giving lectures and sharing his knowledge and skills in treating patients. He has visited 16 countries and regions to lecture.

At present, Hao is developing a purer snake venom injection — the fourth generation — and other medicines. He says: "I want to let the world know that Chinese medical workers are able to develop an effective medicine which can replace surgery."

Yin Hui, a director of the pharmaceutical factory that produces Svate-3, is full of praise for Hao Wenxue. She said: "Prof. Hao has never observed weekends or holidays; he is a complete workaholic."

Hao Wenxue himself says: "Making a little personal sacrifice is worthwhile if my efforts can bring back happiness to many families. I'm old, so I must hurry and try to give more."

FOR RELEVANT ILLUSTRATION, SEE Fig. 1.

CHAPTER 3

A HERBAL INJECTION TO CURE EPILEPSY

Zhao Zhanmin, trained as a surgeon, set out to reduce frequency of epileptic fits by using a plant derivative to improve micro-circulation in the brain. To achieve a swift effect, he uses the injection method to introduce the medicine into the neck artery which carries up to 20 percent of the heart's blood output up to the brain where the problem causing epilepsy is rooted.

Xu Bo is now a normal middle school student just as bright and lively as his classmates, but only a few years ago he was an epileptic unable to walk, speak or care for himself. Things started to go wrong when he was two years old.

Every day he suffered seven or eight epileptic fits. His symptoms shocked his mother and father. He froze like a statue, and other people thought he was mentally-retarded. Desperate for treatment, Xu Bo's distressed parents took him to countless hospitals in Beijing, Shanghai and Tianjin in their quest for a cure — but to no avail.

Then, in the late 1980s, something little short of a miracle occurred. Thanks to herbal medicine injected into his neck he began to show signs of recovery. And over a three-year period of treatment Xu Bo made a full recovery. He has never had a single relapse. But the miraculous treatment was not given in any of the country's leading hospitals. It came from a specialist working at the Epilepsy & Cerebral Disease Hospital in Pinglu County, Shanxi Province.

Dr. Zhao Zhanmin, trained as a surgeon but now a cerebral disease specialist and president of the hospital, recalled that Xu Bo's case took a favorable turn just three days after starting the injection treatment. Soon the boy could take a step. Two days later he could walk 50 meters — unassisted. And after six months of treatment he could speak and walk upstairs and downstairs.

Dr. Zhao, 42, established his epilepsy unit with 32 colleagues in October 1986. With his own herbal injection, Zhao has treated more than 20,000 epileptics and patients with similar brain disorders since 1984. His patients range from babies to pensioners.

New Theory

Epilepsy is a disease of the brain which causes sudden attacks of uncontrolled violent movement and loss of consciousness. Though fits appear to occur at random, some researchers believe that they are triggered off by shock, extremes in temperature, fever, prolonged mental anxiety and excessive alcohol intake.

It is quite a rare disorder. In China, less than seven per thousand suffer. Though researchers cannot agree on the cause of the illness, many of them believe that the condition is produced by extreme excitation of brain cells.

But Zhao Zhanmin does not subscribe to that theory. He has his own. He holds that — apart from the small number (about 0.2 percent) of epileptics who inherit the problem — the occurrence of epilepsy is related to a disturbance in cerebral micro-circulation: blood flow through blood vessels in the brain. Dr. Zhao emphasizes that in his opinion this disturbance is not caused by extreme excitation of brain cells, as some researchers believe.

When a fit comes on, the patient exhibits extremely distorted movements. The whole body, especially the arms and legs, show violent agitation. The patient's face pales and may even turn purple. "This abnormal facial color indicates a lack of oxygen and blood in the patient's tissues and organs," Zhao explained.

Working from this indicator, Zhao further deduced that the spasmodic contraction of the brain's blood vessels during a convulsion could cause a disturbance in cerebral micro-circulation and in turn a lack of oxygen and blood in the brain's membranes. Hence the discoloration of the epileptic's face.

Oral administration of *diazepam valium*, *phenobarbital* and *phenytoin sodium* are conventional treatments for epilepsy. Although these anti-epileptic and sedative medicines reduce over-excitation of brain cells, they have side effects. Patients are likely to acquire deteriorated mentality in the form of slow thinking, reactions and aphasia — speech defects.

After graduating from Yuncheng Medical School in Shanxi and becoming a surgeon in 1975, Zhao was determined to find a new method of treating epilepsy, but without the side effects.

In the course of his library research he came across an article suggesting that a derivative from the henbane family of plants (*Hyoscyamus*) could improve micro-circulation. This was a revelation to Zhao and in 1980 he began to look to the world of plants for a cure for epilepsy. And after much laboratory testing involving 34 stages he produced a pale-yellow liquid extracted from henbane-like plants. He called it Compound Henbane Injection.

Experiments

Between May and July 1984, Zhao used Compound Henbane Injection in 68 experiments conducted on 13 rabbits. He observed that the injection speeded and increased the discharge of blood flow, reduced agglutination of red blood cells while strengthening and increasing the elasticity of blood vessel walls within the brain.

Finally, Zhao induced epilepsy in all 13 rabbits. Those without treatment by injection suffered longer convulsions and the spasms of their blood vessels were more severe than the rabbits given the henbane compound. The convulsions of the injected rabbits appeared to be brought under control within three to five minutes, and their brain micro-circulation improved.

Encouraged by these findings, Zhao began his clinical treatment of patients suffering epilepsy and its sequelae, or complications.

Pharmacological Explanation

Most patients suffered no more epileptic fits after one or two injections, Zhao noted. Since those experimental years, Zhao has perfected his given course of treatment. The initial course lasts 12 days. Six months later, patients undergo two follow-on courses to ensure complete recovery.

Why is Zhao's treatment so fast-acting? The answer lies in its method of administration. Epilepsy is a condition focused in the brain, but the brain only receives 16-20 percent of the heart's total blood output. Hence only a small amount of medicine given orally or by intramuscular injection actually reaches the problem area, the brain, through general circulation.

To sidestep this problem, Zhao drew on his surgical experience. He knew that in any emergency surgical situation, injections should be given in the neck to achieve a quick result. So he decided that his herbal compound should probably be injected there too.

Zhao chose the neck artery — the only direct path taking blood from the heart to the brain — to give his injection. Only in this way, he says, can powerful medicine be carried swiftly and in full to the place where it is needed, and get to work.

According to Zhao, the injection dosage varies according to the patient's condition and age. Some patients have to take *Tongweiling* Capsules, also compounded by Zhao, in addition to the Compound Henbane Injection.

All patients under Zhao's care are told to cease taking previously prescribed medicines. Then the injected herbal medicine can act fully without reaction with other drugs. Its purpose is to dilate the brain's blood vessels, strengthen them and relieve brain membranes from lack of oxygen and blood. The result is no fits, or shorter, less traumatic convulsions.

Fifty-four-year-old Shen Shuxin, a staff member of an agricultural school, first had an epileptic fit in 1983. After that he suffered from attacks once every few months. His condition worsened in 1989 with the fit frequency becoming daily. Dr. Zhao's treatment came to the rescue. Two weeks after his first course of injections in June 1989 he found relief.

"Every morning," Shen recalled, "I was given a 12ml injection in the neck artery. The needle hurt a bit. Once injected, my face felt a little hot. Three to five minutes later, I felt dizzy, then I fell asleep. But I felt great when I woke up."

Ten other patients interviewed reported similar sensations to Shen's and agreed that the injection treatment was effective and induced no noticeable side effects.

Of the 20,000 or more treated epileptics and other patients with various cerebral diseases, follow-up visits have been made on 12,000 patients who had hospital treatment more than three years ago. Statistics concerning these patients show that they have an overall improvement rate of 95.18 percent and that the condition of more than 70 percent of them is completely under control, that is, their fit frequency has been cut by more than 75 percent.

Problems Discussed

While recognizing the curative effect of Zhao's treatment of epileptics, some doctors are skeptical that it is free from side effects.

Fei Yaxin, a neurologist at Beijing Union Hospital, said repeated jabs in the neck artery could damage the vital passageway by which blood reaches the brain. She said that in the worst scenario such puncturing could lead to clotting in the brain blood vessels.

But Zhao says that in his treatment of epileptic patients, bruised arteries are not a problem. However, precautions are taken. His doctors use cotton wool to press the perforation for five or six minutes to ensure that the neck artery is always left intact. Besides, notes Zhao, if some patients do suffer slight bruising, it can easily be soothed by pressing a cold towel against the affected part for about 30 minutes.

Despite the excellent results he has recorded, Zhao continues to strive for improvement. He has recently developed a new herbal extract, to be taken orally, and has been prescribing a number of new, domestically produced Western medicines to accompany his course of herbal injections. As a result, the injection method has become safer and more effective.

In March 1992, Zhao organized the construction of a modern hospital able to accommodate more than 200 patients. It is dedicated to the treatment of epileptics and patients with complications of encephalitis, meningitis and cerebral injuries.

Such dedication to relieve sufferers of epilepsy has not gone unnoticed. In recognition of his contributions to medical science, the Shanxi provincial government has cited Zhao Zhanmin as a model citizen, an outstanding talent and a young expert. And he was elected a deputy to the Provincial People's Congress.

Not surprisingly, news of his effective treatment has spread far and wide. Patients from a dozen foreign countries have visited his hospital for advice and cures. Medical personnel from 36 hospitals, many in remote regions, have contacted Zhao in the hope of studying his methods and introducing them to their own hospitals. "This can be arranged, provided that they're up to standard and that suitably qualified personnel undergo training at our hospital," said Dr. Zhao Zhanmin.

CHAPTER 4

FORGOTTEN POINTS OF ACUPUNCTURE

What do arrowheads, swords and hooks have in common? Primitive weapons yes, but they also describe acupuncture needles rarely used since ancient times. Shi Huaitang has redesigned them, and by applying them with other stimuli, such as heat and magnetism, has created the most comprehensive and widely applicable range of acupuncture treatment available.

Though acupuncture, the unique form of Chinese medicine, has spread around the world, few of its adherents are aware that the commonly-used needle, the capillary needle, was just one of nine used in ancient times.

The earliest Chinese medicine classic written two millennium ago, *The Yellow Emperor's Internal Classic*, describes the nine needles as differing in size and length and having the ability to cure different ailments. Selecting the correct needle was deemed vital: "An appropriate application will cure a chronic disease whereas a poor application will fail to cure."

While most acupuncture practitioners have been content to use just the capillary needle, Shi Huaitang decided early in his career to exhume the long-forgotten use of the other eight instruments of the ancient profession.

It took him 20 years to do that. Since the late 1970s Shi has cured thousands of patients suffering from more than 200 diseases — by using needles of various shapes and sizes.

Revival and Improvement

Now a professor and honorary director of Shanxi Provincial Acupuncture Research Institute in Taiyuan, Shi Huaitang can be regarded as the reviver of New Nine Needle Therapy. But not entirely in the forms used by the ancients.

The 75-year-old doctor invented the plum blossom needle, binding seven needles together, and added it to the old collection. He also amalgamated the ancient long needle with the capillary needle, transformed the sharp needle into a hooked one, and changed the large needle into a fire one. And he also adapted the traditionally used burner for heating the fire needle before applying it.

The ancients used sesame oil, but that left black spots on patients' skin, hence the treatment was never used on the face. Professor Shi discovered that alcohol is a safe fuel, so he uses that in his burners.

Altogether Shi's new nine needles actually comprise ten types and one burner. They are: *Chanzhen* (arrowhead needle), *Ciyuan Meizhen* (round and plum-blossom magnetic percussive-punctator), *Dizhen* (blunt needle), *Meihuazhen* (plum blossom needle), *Fenggouzhen* (hooked needle), *Pizhen* (sword-shaped needle), *Yuanlizhen* (round and sharp needle), *Haozhen* (capillary needle), *Huozhen* (fire needle), and *Sanlengzhen* (three-edged needle).

"Their functions are all different," Shi says. "The arrowhead needle is for respiratory diseases while the round and plum-blossom magnetic percussive-punctator is good for skin complaints and varicose veins. And the blunt needle is useful for stopping bleeding and piles."

But really there is a needle for everything, as Professor Shi's casebook can testify.

Zhang Yongxiang, 65, lost the sight of his right eye with glaucoma in July 1996. After treatment at Beijing's Tongren Hospital, the capital's leading eye hospital, Zhang partially regained his eyesight (0.4). But things still looked fuzzy. Poor eyesight in old age was hereditary in Zhang's family, so the doctors at Tongren advised him to have surgery to correct the problem. Zhang was reluctant. He had a liver problem and was worried about his post-operation recovery. Then his son heard about Shi Huaitang and took his father to see the professor.

Patient's View

"The first treatment Shi gave me immediately improved the amount of light reaching my eyes," Zhang recalls. "He jabbed dozens of needles into my head, and left them there for half an hour. When I woke up the next morning, everything was much clearer and there were no double images. I was saved from surgery!"

Shi continued to treat Zhang for a week, and with both encouraged by the the results, they decided to tackle the liver complaint — cirrhosis.

This time the professor adopted the fire needle option, applied to the abdomen. After only three treatments, Zhang was delighted to find that his sickly-grey complexion was starting to normalize as his once-swollen liver began to shrink in size.

"At first I doubted whether needles could really cure me, but now I'm fully confident in Doctor Shi's hands," Zhang says.

To give his patients confidence, Shi always explains how acupuncture works. He says that the internal state of the human body is reflected by a person's exterior appearance.

"With the needles' jabbing on particular acupoints, a series of changes take place underneath, both circulatory and bioelectrical. Hence the vicinity no longer favors the existence of disease."

Cancer cells, for example, are destroyed by high temperature. Working with this in mind Shi set about treating a patient with suspected skin cancer.

The patient, Wang Zuoyu, from Shanxi, recalls his treatment: "I was 62 that year, and had a mole getting bigger and bigger on my right temple. My own doctor recommended surgical removal, but I was a bit worried about that, so I sought Professor Shi."

"Shi heated a sword-shaped needle and a blunt needle on the alcohol burner until they were red hot. Then he used the needles to remove the mole. In about ten minutes it was gone. It wasn't painful at all. There was no need to take any anti-inflammatory tablets afterwards and I went to work the next day as usual. The wound neither swelled nor festered. And I don't even have a scar. No wonder people call Shi a miraculous surgeon!"

For his part, Shi recalls: "The temperature of the needles was about 800 degrees centigrade. That eased the pain and dispensed with the need for anesthesia. I removed the mole with the sword-shaped needle while stopping bleeding with the blunt needle. The wound formed a scab later on. As Wang said, no hospitalization was needed."

Required Skills

Explaining how to handle needles in general, Shi says acupoints — places on the body where the needles should be applied — are essentials to be familiar with. So is *jingluo*, the meridian system composed of channels and collaterals in the body. A system of specific paths for the circulation of blood and *qi* throughout the body, *jingluo* functions to interlink the solid and hollow *zang-fu* organs, the muscles, tendons, bones, and sensory organs, thus making the body a whole.

Additionally, he stresses, qualified acupuncturists should also have a good command of anatomy, even though anatomy belongs in the field of Western medicine. "A traditional Chinese medicine practitioner should be well versed in both Chinese and Western medicine so as to assimilate the advantages of both."

Finally, clinical experience is indispensable, Shi says, for "one needs to improve one's expertise and the design of needles based on practical treatment."

Shi has improved his round and plum blossom magnetic needle ten times over a 14-year period. It can be said to be in a constant state of evolution. It is a "hammer" with the shaft and heads made from aluminum alloy. While one end of the head is as round as millet and named magnetic round needle, the other end, magnetic plum blossom needle, consists of many embedded needle points.

"What is peculiar about the 'hammer' is that inside its head is a permanent magnet containing cobalt, a rare-earth element, of nearly 5,000 gauss (the unit of electromagnetic induction)," Shi says.

The professor points out that magnetism has, from ancient times, been known to have powerful curative effects. He believes himself to be the first to use it in conjunction with acupuncture.

The first patient he treated with the dual therapy had neurodermatitis in the waist and right lower limb. Shi punctured the focuses with his plum blossom needle twice a week. Several months later, the patient's waist condition improved, but the leg did not respond. Shi then experimented by affixing a big magnet on the leg with the aid of a bandage. In two weeks, the leg recovered. This inspired Shi to think about integrating the plum blossom needle with magnetism.

His work was completed in 1978 and the new needle was patented in 1985, as are all the other needles he renovated or developed. It is unique because it can be used by both doctors and ordinary people, as Shi has written a reference guide for the layman.

In contrast, the fire needle, available in five types — fine, medium, rough, hooked, and three-pointed — should only be used by experienced acupuncturists.

Methods of applying the fire needle generally involve pricking that combines hooking, point pricking, deep pricking, shallow pricking, swift insertion, slow insertion, and inserting with the needle remaining at the point for a few seconds, depending on conditions of the cases.

Acupuncture can treat an array of diseases and complaints, but Shi specializes in brandy nose, acne, freckles, warts, varicose veins, bone tuberculosis and underarm odor.

Mi Lanfang, a middle-aged farmer from Xiangfen County, Shanxi Province, contracted bone tuberculosis which paralyzed her in the legs. Despite nearly 200 injections of *streptomycin*, she still could not move. After Shi gave her four treatments with his fire needle and plum blossom needle she was able to walk with the aid of a stick. She went on to recover fully after 20 treatments.

News of such stunning results have spread out from Shi's native Shanxi. Among his VIP patients were senior leaders Liu Shaoqi, Hua Guofeng, Hu Yaobang, and Liu Bocheng.

Students from 24 countries have attended Shi's acupuncture class in Yuncheng, his home town. And he has lectured in the United States, Singapore and South Korea. He estimates he has taught some 10,000 students of acupuncture, with his New Nine Needle Therapy being practiced clinically throughout China and in more than 20 other countries and regions.

Despite this, Shi is worried that his expertise cannot be fully passed on to the next generation. "Few young people in China have the diligence or patience to master the New Nine Needle Therapy. They are eager to make money. To me spreading the ancient therapy is a more important cause. It is a valuable heritage that was once lost for 2,000 years. It should never be lost again."

FOR RELEVANT ILLUSTRATIONS, SEE Figs. 2-6.

CHAPTER 5

TAKING THE PAIN OUT OF CONQUERING THE BIG C

An emulsion extracted from a grass indigenous to South China equals and sometimes betters conventional cancer treatments while inducing virtually no side effects. Its formulation was the result of more than 17 years' dedicated lab work during which time Li Dapeng, the inventor of Kanglaite, nearly lost his own life in the course of experimentation.

With the improvement of a variety of chemically-synthesized anti-tumor drugs and chemotherapy in recent years, those diagnosed as having cancer need not regard the news as synonymous to receiving the death sentence. If detected and treated sooner, rather than later, the big C can be the little c.

Although differing degrees of recovery are commonly being brought about, patients generally have to endure much pain and trauma during their long courses of treatment in which various side effects, such as hair-loss and chronic nausea, manifest themselves. Liver, kidney and bone marrow functions are particularly susceptible to imbalance when the body is exposed to powerful chemically-synthesized medicines.

Traditional Chinese medicines, on the other hand, comprising naturally-occurring materials, are valued for their purity as alternatives with few or no side effects. But generally they tend to be more useful as preventative rather than curative medicines.

One exception to this general rule, however, is an anti-tumor medicine called *Kanglaite*. It is derived from the seeds of a grass found in South China.

"For years, we have been searching for a Chinese medicine that not only fortifies health, but also combats cancer," says Xu Guangwei, director of the Beijing Tumor Hospital. "We're glad this dream has come true."

"*Kanglaite* is effective, but with few side effects. So patients find it acceptable," comments Wu Liangcun, a cancer specialist and former administrator at the Traditional Chinese Medicine Hospital of Zhejiang Province. He was responsible for overseeing clinical trials on *Kanglaite* in the late 1980s.

Case Histories

Wu recalled a recent case, that of Xiao Aiyun, 61. She attended hospital in April 1996, her eyes and body yellow and itching. The sickly color was tell-tale of a chronic liver problem. Indeed, X-ray pictures confirmed this: her liver was swollen, and a focus, 6.6 x 8cm, could be seen. The adjacent organ, the pancreas, could not be detected. It was hidden by the cancerous growth within the liver.

Xiao was prescribed three 100ml bottles of *Kanglaite*. The medicine is injected — a unique method of administering Chinese medicine — thus enabling it to reach the diseased area quickly via circulation in the bloodstream.

An examination several months after Xiao's treatment found the focus to be half its original size — 4 x 3.3cm. And her complexion was gradually returning to normal.

Pan Chaobo, from China's southeastern Zhejiang Province, suffered from primary liver cancer. He was desperate after chemotherapy by intravenous drip proved virtually ineffective. Hearing of the *Kanglaite* injection, he decided to have a try. In December 1992 at the age of 36, he received arterial perfusions of 100ml per dose per week for two successive weeks. This was complemented by a course of treatment by intravenous drip (100ml per day), which lasted for 20 days.

Two months later, the focus had reduced in size to 7 x 9cm from its original 17 x 19cm.

CONQUERING THE BIG C • 27

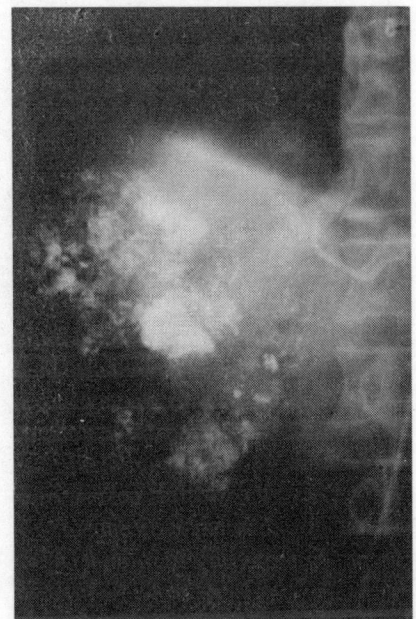

X-ray of Pan Chaobo's liver cancer, before treatment.

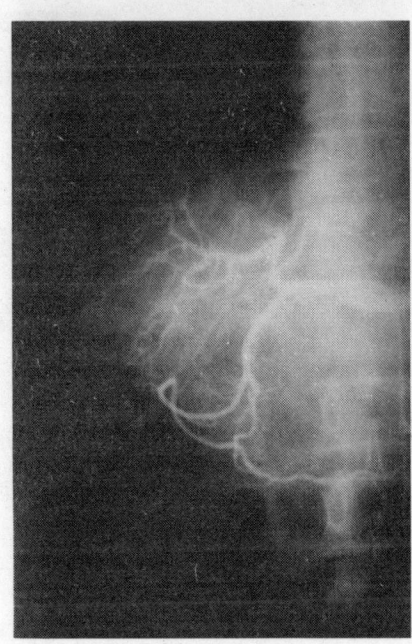

X-ray of the liver after treatment. Pan, now 42, leads a normal life since being treated with *Kanglaite* injections five years ago.

28 • UNBELIEVABLE CURES AND MEDICINES

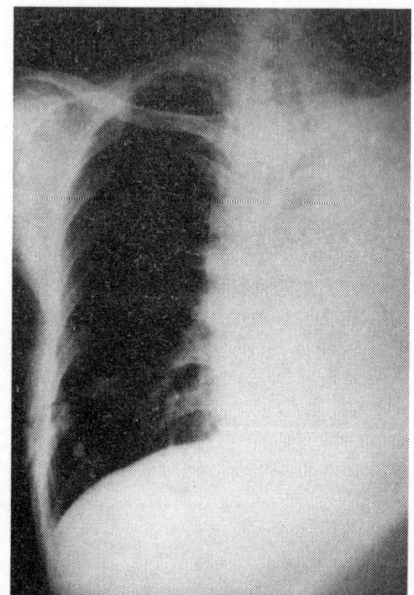

X-ray of Wang Xiaowu's lung cancer, before treatment.

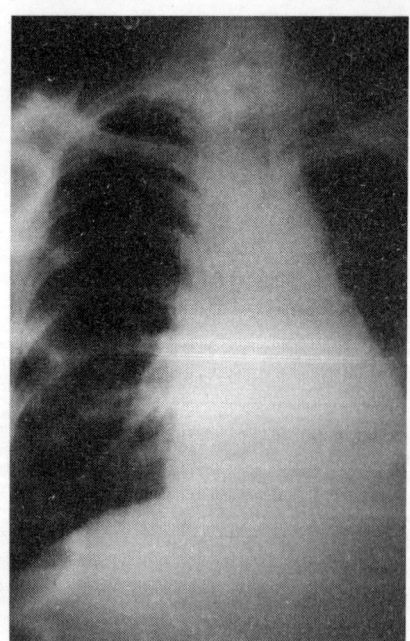

X-ray of the lung after treatment. Wang, now 61, had *Kanglaite* injections four years ago.

Terminal Patients Cured

Soon after *Kanglaite*'s formulation, it underwent clinical testing on terminal cancer patients. They were willing to try the medication as a last resort: they had no other way to turn. Doctors had predicted the patients would only live for days or weeks, months at the most.

Doctors had to swallow their words. Today (mid-1997), more than 90 percent of those patients, the first group to ever benefit from *Kanglaite*, are alive.

How does it work?

Pharmacodynamic research, which explores the reaction between drugs and living systems, shows that the medicine induces a similar "killing" effect on certain cancer cells as do chemically-synthesized drugs.

Clinical trials show that *Kanglaite* injection can lead to extensive necrosis of the tumor's surface. In this way, cancer cells are inhibited or killed, and the spread and metastasis of cancer cells contained.

To date, *Kanglaite* injections have been used clinically in China, Australia, Germany, Indonesia, Japan, Britain, the United States and Hong Kong in treating nearly 10,000 patients. It has achieved noteworthy results.

Furthermore, compared with synthesized drugs, *Kanglaite* does not damage healthy white blood cells, but instead promotes blood-generating and immunological functions.

Kanglaite and *Taoxl* Compared

Trials show *Kanglaite* to be more effective than *Taoxl* for treating lung and liver cancer. *Taoxl*, widely used, took 25 years' research and approximately US$2 billion in funding to develop. But unlike *Taoxl*, which quite commonly causes aches and allergies, *Kanglaite* induces virtually no side effects.

Whereas *Taoxl* achieves best results when prescribed for gynecological tumors, *Kanglaite* is efficacious for a larger scope of cancers from embryonic to advanced stages, particularly primary lung cancer, liver cancer, colon cancer, gastric carcinoma, throat cancer, kidney cancer, malignant lymph tumor and leukemia.

Authoritative clinical data shows that, even in treating gynecologic tumors, the effectiveness of *Kanglaite* is only seven percentage points lower than *Taoxl*'s 57 percent.

Chemotherapy is regarded as the inevitable course of treatment for late cancer sufferers. But clinical trials show that the effective rate of *Kanglaite* is 20.6 percent, approaching that of chemotherapy, which is 25.2 percent.

Chemotherapy's side effects are feared by patients and relatives alike. Hair loss, nausea, and hematopoietic disorder, a bone marrow problem, are common occurrences. Chemotherapy also kills large quantities of white blood cells, leaving patients debilitated.

Kanglaite, on the contrary, does not induce such horrific side effects; it actually improves the performance of those useful cells and increases the number of white blood cells.

A comparative trial showed that 10 out of 11 patients undergoing chemotherapy recorded reduced white blood counts. But when the same patients were treated with *Kanglaite*, only 1 in 6 suffered from a reduced count.

An additional *Kanglaite* property is that it is a source of nutrition, being a medicine based on a plant extract. It provides three times more energy per unit volume than the 10% glucose fluid commonly used in IV-drips. Therefore it is ideal for weak, middle- and late-stage cancer patients who suffer from low energy levels.

Kanglaite can be administered either independently or as a complementary preparation at the same time as chemotherapy, radiotherapy or biotherapy.

"*Kanglaite* is a successful combination of traditional Chinese medicine and advanced techniques", according to Wu Jieping, one of China's leading medical experts and a Chinese Academy of Sciences (CAS) member.

Extracted from Grass

The medicine contains an active substance extracted from the seeds of Job's Tears (*Coix Lachryma Jobi*) — a common grass found in damp areas, especially along river banks and valleys of southern China.

Its usefulness in combating a host of ailments and diseases has long been recognized and recorded. The slightly-sweet-tasting seed is well known for easing cramp and alleviating fatigue. Besides, it can also function as a sedative and pain-killer. Seeds of Job's Tears have traditionally been valued for their effectiveness in curing appendicitis, pulmonary abscesses, diarrhea, and gastric problems.

Li Dapeng, the man behind *Kanglaite*, recalls the first time he thought of conducting research on Job's Tears seeds. "Twenty years ago, when I was reading a Japanese medical journal, I learned that scientists in that country were trying to derive an extract by boiling Job's Tears seeds."

But he noted they were not making much progress, and their methods were proving too expensive.

Li, a graduate from Shanghai Medical University, was interested in separating the derivative himself. But he had to find a way where the Japanese had failed.

He knew that a long, hard road of research lay ahead. But underlying his determination to succeed was a genuine belief in the purity of traditional Chinese medicine, Li's main field of interest, even though he had majored in Western medicine. However, even at this early stage, he wanted to derive an extract from the miraculous seeds and introduce it by injection — a Western method — into the human body. Most Chinese medicines are taken orally or applied externally.

The advantage of the injecting method is that the active substance contained therein can be fully absorbed through blood circulation and directed by it, swiftly, to the focus.

Research Outset

Li's basic research on *Kanglaite* and the injection method began in 1976. A decade later, he had separated a white emulsion from the Job's Tears seeds and it underwent preliminary clinical testing on terminal patients who had been told they had no hope of recovery.

Li Dapeng, then research chief at the Traditional Chinese Medicine Hospital of Zhejiang Province, had only received the equivalent of approximately US$5,000 in funding from the government, and was actually putting his own money into his research. Hindered by the shortage of finance, Li was forced to embark on a fund-raising program. Eventually he collected US$2.17 million for further work.

But his worries were not over. In 1989, while experimenting in an unventilated basement room, his apparatus exploded. With sixty-five percent of his skin severely burnt, he was rushed to hospital with his life in the balance. But Li recovered, put this disaster behind him, and resumed his work.

In June, 1993, *Kanglaite* was recognized as a scientific research achievement by the State Administration of Traditional Chinese Medicine. In 1995, almost 20 years after research began, *Kanglaite* injection received patents in both China and the United States. Applications have also been made in ten other countries.

Dr. Li Dapeng is now chairman of the board of the Hangzhou-based Zhejiang *Kanglaite* Pharmaceutical Co., Ltd. which is devoted to the research and manufacture of the cancer-fighting injection. The company's factory began producing the drug in November, 1995. In its first year of operation it produced 80,000 bottles.

FOR RELEVANT ILLUSTRATIONS, SEE Figs. 7 & 8.

CHAPTER 6

A DEADLY WEED: MEDICINE IN MEDICAL HANDS

Ba Bu Dao, the name of a seemingly deadly-poisonous plant found in China's central and southern uplands, is also a warning. It means "drop dead after eight steps." But the danger is only superficial: the root sap of this vine is the main ingredient of a medicine that has given mobility back to thousands stiffened with rheumatoid arthritis.

A disaster befell Teng Yongli one morning as she was having breakfast. Her fingers just seized up. But before she tried to fathom out the reason why, she asked herself "How will I be able to play the piano?"

Teng's livelihood and love were soon in jeopardy as the mobility of slender, delicate fingers disappeared. She had an enjoyable and promising profession, being employed as a teacher and musician at the Central Conservatory of Music in Beijing.

The diagnosis, when it came, was a shock: rheumatoid arthritis.

Slowly the complaint crept through her entire body. Soon she was confined to her home, let alone did she have the finger sensitivity required to play her favorite pieces of Chopin and Tchaikovsky.

"I thought I was done for," she recalls. "So I took whatever medicine I came across — but none of it worked."

In 1990, Teng's husband, a journalist, brought her yet another bottle of tablets and asked her to try them. They were new, he said, and might work.

Teng took them, but expected no miracle. Yet to her amazement, she felt better shortly afterwards. Swellings began to subside, stiffness and pain gradually eased. "After taking six bottles of the tablets in two months, I was able to stand up and go shopping with my husband," she says.

Teng, now 53, leads a normal life. Her fingers, though not as delicate as when she was young, are nimble enough to play the world's great piano pieces again.

Root of Recovery

The woman is one of hundreds of thousands who have benefited from a drug called *Triptergium Multiglycoside*. It is extracted from a deadly poisonous herb, *Triptergium Wilfordii* in Latin and known as *Lei Gong Teng* in Chinese. It grows mainly in mountainous areas of central and southern China.

Lei Gong Teng, or "thunder god vine," is also known as *Ba Bu Dao* — literally warning that anyone who takes it by mistake will drop dead after eight steps. Farmers in some areas use its sap as a natural pesticide on vegetables.

In 1973, a group of researchers from the Nanjing-based Chinese Academy of Medical Sciences began tapping the medicinal values of the deadly weed. This followed the reported success of doctors of traditional Chinese medicine in Fujian Province, East China, who had used decoctions of the herb's root sap to treat rheumatoid arthritis.

The team was led by Prof. Lu Xieyu of the academy's Dermatology Institute, an expert in extracting substances with medicinal value from herbs.

In 1978, Prof. Lu and his colleagues succeeded in extracting a substance from *Triptergium Wilfordii* roots, which they named *Triptergium Multiglycoside*. After conducting extensive pharmacological and toxicological experiments on rats, dogs and other animals, the researchers concluded that the substance had significant anti-inflammatory and immuno-suppressive properties.

In October 1979, Tripterium Multiglycoside-TII-14 in tablet form was given clearance for trial use. This was followed by clinical experiments conducted between 1981-82 in 18 hospitals across the country, including some of China's best known institutions, such as the Beijing Union Hospital, General Hospital of the People's Liberation Army of Nanjing Military Area Command and Wuxi Hospital of Traditional Chinese Medicine.

First Trials

A total of 554 patients diagnosed as suffering from various diseases were chosen for treatment with *Triptergium Multiglycoside*. The length of each administered course varied from case to case, from 10 days to three months. "It was as long as seven months in some rare cases," Prof. Lu said.

The patients were grouped according to their complaints as follows: 144 with rheumatoid arthritis; 116 with skin diseases; 114 with kidney disease; 57 with leprosy-B, 54 with hepatitis, 51 with *mucositis* of the oral cavity (ulcers); 15 with systematic *lupus erythematosus* (a skin complaint); and three with other diseases. Each patient took a daily dose of 1-1.5mg for each kilogram of his or her body weight.

The medicine proved particularly effective in dealing with rheumatoid arthritis and skin diseases, with 93.3 and 94.6 percent of the treated patients showing varying degrees of improvement. The rates for "marked improvement" were recorded at 55.1 and 79 percent respectively.

In the treatment of hepatitis and systematic *lupus erythematosus*, performances of 66.6 percent effectivity and 33.3 percent marked effectivity were recorded.

Summarizing, Prof. Lu says that "patients' symptoms were gone or alleviated by their completion of courses."

What is remarkable about the medicine is that "it achieves good results when used to treat some diseases of unknown origins — systematic *lupus erythematosus* and *mucositis* of the oral cavity," Prof. Lu says.

Systematic *lupus erythematosus* is a slowly progressive systemic disorder characterized by inflammation of the skin. Western medicine provides no sure cure for it. *Mucositis* of the oral cavity, or simply mouth ulcers, causes great pain to patients but is quite harmless.

Effective Component

In 1982, *Triptergium Multiglycoside* passed state appraisal, and later came to be listed as a basic medicine in *China Pharmacopoeia*. But researchers were still baffled by this question: since *Triptergium Multiglycoside* is a multi-elemental substance, which element is medically effective?

Work continued on *Triptergium Multiglycoside* and, in 1987, Lu and his colleagues identified tripchlorolide, a chemical compound in the herb, as being the medically effective substance in *Triptergium Multiglycoside*.

"Undoubtedly, this is a poisonous type of medicine," Lu says. "But like snake poison, it can be used to attack some inveterate diseases if good control is exercised in its application. As a matter of fact, use of one type of poison to eliminate poison of another type is part of the theory and practice of traditional Chinese medicine."

Clinical use has indicated that the medicine induces a side effect. It can lower white blood cell counts in some patients. Such patients are advised to cease using the drug temporarily until blood testing shows normalized white-red blood count ratios.

Mass production of the medicine started in 1989, even though one ton of the herb yields only a few grams of the medically effective substance.

Zhejiang DND Pharmaceutical Co. Ltd., a state owned company in Xinchang, Zhejiang Province, manufactures the drug. "We chose to produce the medicine mainly because of the rich resources of *Triptergium Wilfordii* in our province," says Jin Zhanghong, general manager of the enterprise.

In 1995, the company turned out 100 kilograms of *Triptergium Multiglycoside*, or 100 million tablets, four times it's first year's production.

The Ministry of Public Health has given the green light for the medicine's export, Jin says, adding that it has already been exported to Germany, Sri Lanka and India.

"We have been inundated by mail from all over the country," he says. "Some are thank-you letters from patients cured by the medicine, others ask for a sample of the medicine to try."

An estimated four million Chinese are suffering from rheumatoid arthritis and systematic *lupus erythematosus*. "Worldwide, the number is much greater," Jin says. "We feel it is a rewarding undertaking to be able to do something to relieve the sufferings of such patients, no matter where they are."

FOR RELEVANT ILLUSTRATIONS, SEE Figs. 9 & 10.

CHAPTER 7

THE POINT OF HEAT

You Fushan is one of the main revivers of fire needle therapy, the long-dormant practice of heating an acupuncture needle to a high temperature before insertion. But it's not as simple as that; the skill rests with the practitioner's ability in choosing the correct needle, inserting it to the optimum depth, and much more.

The practitioner holds a small alcohol burner in his left hand and an acupuncture needle in his right. Heated until it glows, the needle is pricked around the ankle of a sportsman who has an overuse injury. He grimaces time and time again. But once the treatment is concluded he walks away, confident of being able to train.

This treatment, known as fire needle, combines acupuncture and heat and can deal with hundreds of common injuries and stubborn diseases.

One type of China's traditional acupuncture therapies, the fire needle was already widely used more than 2,000 years ago, according to ancient Chinese medical classics. Over the centuries, however, its use was abandoned, probably because of difficulties encountered in preparing the needles correctly, not to mention the complexities of the operation itself.

As a result, treatment by fire needle has been experienced by a relatively small number of people. *The Illustrated Dictionary of Chinese Acupuncture*, published in 1978, referred to the procedure as "obsolete."

Although few fire needle practitioners can be found in China now, the ancient technique is certainly not extinct. A handful of practitioners are making enthusiastic efforts to revive the dormant therapy. One of the prime movers is You Fushan, a doctor who has established a fire needle clinic in Gansu Province, northwest China.

Dr. You, 45, has been applying this therapy during his 20 years of clinical practice and successfully treated more than 56,000 patients afflicted with such diseases as bone tuberculosis, rheumatic arthritis, bone spurs, paralysis, asthma, some chronic stomach troubles, and armpit odor. He claims that the fire needle therapy can also prevent hepatitis and some other infectious diseases.

Case Studies

The doctor has applied the fire needle therapy for cosmetic purposes. In 1993, a famous Hong Kong film star felt depressed at the appearance of a small facial growth. When she learned that fire needle therapy could remove it, she tried every means to seek out Dr. You, who was then lecturing in Shanxi Province. She told the doctor that she did not care how much the treatment cost, so long as it could remove the nevus and leave no scar. He did just that for her.

An engineer from Russia suffered for years from the embarrassment of *hircismus* — unpleasant armpit odor. When he came to Dr. You, the doctor sterilized and anesthetized the region to be treated before heating a specially-shaped, three-pronged needle over an alcohol burner until it was red-hot. He then punctured the armpits at key points. After that, he used a thicker needle, one millimeter in diameter, to prick the roots of the hair follicles and open the sweat sacs, draining the fluid. Finally he applied *erythromycin* cream to the pinpricks and bandaged the area. In just a few minutes the "surgery" was done and the patient was cured of his complaint.

A more serious case involved a worker, Zhang Xiuying, a 42-year-old from Lanzhou. She was diagnosed with a form of tuberculosis afflicting her spine in 1991. She went from hospital to hospital seeking a cure, but to no avail. The skin in the area had turned black and her spine had become so distended that she couldn't straighten her back. She could no longer do her work.

Then she heard of Dr. You's fire needle therapy. After two months of treatment at his clinic, the skin covering the afflicted region had healed, and an X-ray examination showed that the affected joints had begun to calcify anew. Now she can straighten her back again and is able to perform household chores.

Dr. You has also applied the fire needle treatment to bone spurs with "quite satisfactory" results. In 1994 and 1995 alone, he cured more than 2,000 patients who had been suffering from spurs in various forms.

Bone spur, known as hyperosteogeny in Western medical science, is a common but hard-to-cure complaint in the middle-aged and elderly. Many sufferers feel such acute pain that they even lose their ability to work. To tackle this problem, Dr. You invented a special fire needle.

He first dresses the area to be treated with ointment, prepared by himself, to soften the overgrown bone tissues. Then he cuts off the spur with his fire needle. Finally he applies some Chinese medicine to that part of the body to hasten the digestion and absorption of the spur inside the body.

The minutes-long "surgery" is performed with accuracy and with a minimum amount of pain. In July, 1994, Dr. You demonstrated this therapy at an international acupuncture seminar in Lanzhou. The "operation" drew much attention from both Chinese and foreign participants.

Needle Types

The doctor attributes his successes to both his thorough knowledge of acupuncture techniques and to the salutary effects of the heated needles. Most acupuncturists use only capillary needles, which are generally made of gold, silver or stainless steel, with handles of bronze or aluminum. In Chinese, these needles are known as *Gan Zhen*, or stem needles. While the capillary needles only require simple sterilization with a cotton swab dipped in alcohol at room temperature, a fire needle is heated to a temperature approaching 800 degrees centigrade before being inserted into the acupoints. To withstand these extreme temperatures, the needles must be of a molybdenum-wolfram steel alloy.

Traditional Chinese medicine holds that fire needle therapy warms the body's channels and collaterals, promoting blood circulation by removing blood stasis and quickening the metabolism. The positive effects include a more resistant immune system and a reduction of dampness, coldness and soreness. The technique also speeds the expulsion and replacement of dead and worn-out tissues.

Miraculous Pivot, one of the two parts of *The Yellow Emperor's Internal Classic*, presents the fundamentals of acupuncture as it was practiced during the Warring States Period (475-221BC). At that time, fire needle acupuncture was generally known as *Fan Zhen*. According to the classic, it was used to treat such maladies as tuberculous cervical lymphadenitis, abdominal cysts and tumors. It became known as *Huo Zhen*, or fire needle, only after the Ming Dynasty was established in 1368.

Originally, fire needles were made of a kind of rough, mottled iron. The choice of material was largely dictated by a folk belief that iron could combat pathogenic elements. The ancient fire needles were 10 to 12cm long and had round, thick bodies some two millimeters in diameter. The points were very sharp, and the handles were made from animal horn or bamboo. Since the needles resembled those used to stitch shoes, they came to be known as *Xie Zhen*, or shoe needles. Along with the evolution of the technique, bronze and copper were used, and finally there came the alloy needles.

The success of the therapy was said to depend on the depth of insertion. If too deep, the channels would be injured, and if too shallow, the treatment would have no effect. This was the assessment of Huangfu Mi, a scholar of the Three Kingdoms Period (220-280) and a native of Gansu's Lingtai County, who compiled *The A-B Classic of Acupuncture and Moxibustion*, the earliest systematic work on acupuncture and moxibustion extant in China.

The heat source for the ancient fire needle was pure sesame oil. After an oil lamp was filled with the liquid, the fire needle was heated over the flame. A newly-made fire needle would be heated for a continuous 24 hours, to anneal it. Then it could be used for treatment. A fire needle master would always reheat the needle until it turned white hot before piercing the focus or acupoints, to sterilize it and achieve the desired effect. Obviously, this primitive needle and heating process was troublesome for both the fire needle practitioner and the patient subjected to the treatment.

That is where Dr. You has improved the technique. He learned how to apply the fire needle therapy from his grandfather when he was still a teenager. Later, he studied with the nine-needle expert Shi

Huaitang, gaining proficiency through years of practice. He has refined and perfected his skill, and made innovations.

Innovations

For instance, to reduce the needle heating time, he replaced the sesame oil lamp with an alcohol burner. To minimize the pain patients have to endure during treatment, he made the steel needles very thin. On discovering that the stainless steel needle tended to bend easily on heating, he developed fire needles made of molybdenum-wolfram alloy steel. To treat different ailments, each of which requires insertion of the needles to different depths, he developed ten types of fire needles, each of a particular thickness, length and shape.

For most treatments, fire needles 0.4 to 1.0 millimeters in diameter are used. In other cases — such as to remove nevus and senile plaque, or to treat superficial infections caused by skin diseases, skin cancer, or *hircismus* — three-pronged fire needles are used. For herpes, warts and flatwarts, and for hyperosteogeny and anal piles, two different kinds of needles are used. Dr. You has also developed other types of fire needles for scraping.

"To be a modern fire needle master," says Dr. You, "the basic thing is to know and master the diagnostic theory of traditional Chinese medicine, namely the 'four diagnostic methods.' That is a general term covering techniques of inspection, auscultation and olfaction, interrogation, taking the pulse and palpation. In addition, the modern acupuncturist must become proficient in identifying, mixing and prescribing medicinal herbs and drugs. It is also important to advance theories and practices of traditional Chinese medicine with reference to modern medical practices."

Dr. You emphasizes that his fire needle therapy combines insights in traditional Chinese medicine and Western medicine. A skilled practitioner of fire needle techniques must make the right choice of acupoints and needles, and must know how to precisely manipulate the needles, while closely monitoring the needle temperature. To treat different diseases, the acupuncturist must sometimes make decisions on the spot, which requires both quick thinking and flexibility. There are many crucial considerations which must be taken into account, such as the selection of acupoints, the depth to which the needle should be inserted, the speed at which it is inserted, and the thickness of the needle to be used.

One form of needle manipulation is called the "flying method." Following the insertion, the needle is rotated in one direction, and when resistance is felt, the needle is released suddenly, creating a light vibration. The sudden releasing action causes the acupuncturist's fingers to resemble the spread wings of a bird, hence the term "flying."

The skillful manipulation of the needle is a key to effect the cure. To treat rheumatism and bone tuberculosis, needles are inserted to a greater depth than for less serious maladies. They are either inserted into prescribed acupoints, or circling the focus. Sometimes patients receive an auxiliary treatment, such as cupping. This is a method of applying a cup in which a partial vacuum is created over an acupoint. The external application of herbal medicines and the use of electromagnetic therapy can accelerate the healing process and strengthen the therapeutic effect.

To test new techniques for the treatment of different diseases with the fire needles, Dr. You has experimented on himself thousands of times. His research and practice have been fruitful: he has published over ten academic papers in China, and has also written a book entitled *Basic Knowledge of Traditional Chinese Medicine* and *the Clinical Application of Fire Needles*, which has been published and distributed by the Lanzhou University Publishing House.

A medical delegation from South Africa showed great interest in Dr. You's fire needle therapy during their visit to Lanzhou and expressed the wish that he could make a lecture tour to their country. "It seems that there are opportunities to extend this special treatment which is part of the treasure house of traditional Chinese medicine," says the doctor, adding that he is optimistic about the future of this ancient healing art. "I, for one, will try my best to further perfect the fire needle technique."

FOR RELEVANT ILLUSTRATION, SEE Fig. 11.

CHAPTER 8

PUTTING ANTS TO WORK ON ARTHRITIS

What contains vitamins B_1, B_2 and E, 28 different amino acids and zinc? Some multivitamin pills of course. But ants from mountainous Guangxi, a region of south China, also do, naturally. Dr. Wu Zhicheng has devoted his career to recruiting billions of these creepy-crawlies for medical work against rheumatoid arthritis, thus writing a fascinating postscript to the 2,000-year-long history of Chinese practitioners valuing the curative powers of ants.

He is known among his patients as "Mr. Ant," a nickname that directly spells out his special field. For this man uses ants to relieve patients of painful joint swellings, symptomatic of rheumatism — one of the world's most common immobilizing diseases that torments millions of people.

His real name is Wu Zhicheng and he's the only expert in China known for his consistent and systematic study in treating diseases, particularly rheumatism, with ants. After 40 years of research and practice, he has perfected methods of using ants to make medicines.

More than 50,000 patients suffering from rheumatoid arthritis are recovering under his prescriptions. Among them, more than 5,000 people who were once paralyzed attribute their miraculous recoveries to the properties of medicine containing the tiny insects.

"Compared with chemical compounds, ant medicines have a prolonged effect on the patient and are unlikely to cause side effects," Mr. Ant claims.

Gao Yuefang, a female worker in her 40s from Henan Province, is always willing to tell her tale of recovery. Paralyzed after a four-year-long battle with rheumatoid arthritis, she almost lost hope and the will to live. As a last resort she took some "ant powder."

Surprisingly, her symptoms began to subside within five days, and two months later her once-stiff fingers could move. "How I longed to stand up again and lead the life of a healthy person! Now I have some hope," she says.

Rheumatism afflicts plagues 0.4 to 3 percent of the world's population. In China, its incidence is about 0.6 percent. In Western medicine, the disease was first diagnosed in 1858 by a Briton, but its cause remains unclear and an effective cure is still the dream of the majority of its sufferers.

Ant Composition

Ants can work wonders because their chemical make-up resembles a counter in a health store. According to Wu, some species of mountain ants contain 40 to 50 percent protein, 28 kinds of free amino acids (eight of which are essential to the human body), vitamins B_1, B_2 and E, as well as many other beneficial minerals and chemical compounds.

These substances contained in ants are listed as being essential to the cure of the rheumatoid disease, according to traditional Chinese medicine theories. The theories diagnose the disease as "an illness of deficiency," resulting from a malfunction of the kidneys, but weather conditions — wind, chill and damp — which discomfort the person, together with blood circulation and *qi*, or vigor, are also recognized factors.

Ants and their ova made into medicines have proved to be highly effective in building up physical strength, toning up the kidneys and combating effects of cold as well as relaxing muscles and tendons to promote blood circulation.

Ants may also be therapeutic because of their zinc content. Modern theories hold that a lack of the trace element might cause rheumatism. Wu reports that the zinc content of ants ranks first among all animals and plants known today. One kilogram of ants contain 110 to 120 milligrams of zinc. Ants are therefore an excellent zinc source, he says.

Cases show that ant-based medicines, made of ants and other herbs, can relieve pain and swelling when rheumatic arthritis causes the deformation of joints. But it can cure once and for all if the disease is caught and treated at its onset. It often takes three to six months for such early-stage patients to recover.

Wu began to appreciate the value of ants used in medicine from locals in northeast China. In 1948, as an army medic serving in Liaoning Province, he felt helpless seeing so many soldiers wounded in battles and being unable to treat them properly due to a poor supply of medicine. So Wu had to make do with what could be found in the forest and fields. And that included ants.

When told that the decoction of ants could sterilize wounds and eliminate pus, he collected some ants and used them to wash the wounds, as locals directed. He also ground dried ants and mixed the powder with yellow rice or millet wine for wounded soldiers to drink. The result was encouraging: the soldiers' wounds no longer festered and their faces were no longer pale.

Later, when his army swept south, he learnt more about folk methods of treating pulmonary diseases, tuberculosis, some skin diseases and arthritis, in particular with ant medicines.

Long Valued

Wu began to research into the history of ant therapy by consulting ancient medical books. He found that ants had, for centuries, been regarded by the ancients as therapeutic.

In fact, as early as in the Han Dynasty (206BC-220AD), ants were used in the making of *Jingangwan*, a widely-used medicine for the treatment of weak bones and muscles. The effectiveness of ant medicines was also mentioned in Tang Dynasty (618-907) records. Later, Li Shizhen, the great Chinese medical scientist of the 16th century, gave a detailed account of ants' medicinal values in his *Compendium of Materia Medica*.

From these ancient books and his ant-collecting tours in South China, Wu found out that 95 percent of ants can be used to make medicines. The only ants not suitable for medicinal use are yellow ants, foul-smelling ants and environmentally-polluted ants. And though all ants contain a small amount of toxin, that can be rendered inert and harmless by processing.

Based on this knowledge, Wu developed his first ant medicine, a powder, for treating rheumatoid arthritis. To facilitate its efficiency, he later developed an amber-colored ant tonic wine to be drunk with the powder.

The powder has been licensed by the public health authorities of the Chinese army, and is used in military hospitals. It is soon expected to be further approved and licensed by the Ministry of Public Health.

The tonic wine has not only worked for patients. At 60, Wu looks young, has a healthy complexion and strong physique. His secret? Two cups of wine — ant wine of course — every lunchtime before his nap. He calls the wine "youth liquor."

Wu is now working as technical consultant of the Jinling Ant Research & Treatment Center affiliated with the Political Academy of the People's Liberation Army in Nanjing. He is also director of the center's rheumatoid arthritis department. It was established in 1980 for Wu to administer his ant therapy after fellow army doctors recognized the potential of the treatment and considered it "very promising."

Since then, Wu's ant therapy has spread around the country. With backing from his center he has set up rheumatoid arthritis clinics in more than 60 cities. He spends about six months each year touring them, treating patients and training young doctors.

Ant Hunts

The center and the clinics require an average of 250 tons of ants a year (about 20,000 ants weigh one kilogram). Most of the insects are collected from South China's Guangxi Zhuang Autonomous Region, a veritable ant kingdom. Local farmers cash in on the demand for ants by catching, drowning and drying the insects before sending them to Nanjing. All of Wu's suppliers have been personally instructed by him so they collect only the species he requires.

Wu is no longer a medic with only six-years' primary schooling and two-years' training in a military medical school. With a little help from the humble ant he has established a radical cure for rheumatism. And with clinical success behind him, Wu has popularized his ant therapy by writing five medical books, 58 theses and more than 300 articles for medical and scientific journals.

He is now medical consultant of the Chinese Academy of

Traditional Chinese Medicine and the country's leading expert on ant therapy. And of course he has received much recognition, in the form of titles, for his work.

But the title Wu likes best is his nickname: Mr. Ant. He believes it simply and succinctly conveys his special field of practice — and it constantly reminds him of his life's work: using ants to cure those crippled with rheumatoid arthritis.

FOR RELEVANT ILLUSTRATIONS, SEE Figs. 12 & 13.

CHAPTER 9

REMOVING SOURCES OF PAIN WITH THE BLADE-TIPPED NEEDLE

It is certain that medical dictionaries of the future will include the name of Prof. Zhu Hanzhang as the inventor and pioneer of a new type of non-invasive surgery given the name "acupotomy", a word composed of the first five letters of "acupoint" and the last four of "anatomy". Etymologically it relates the combined nature of the instrument, part surgical scalpel part acupuncture needle, and aptly called a "needle-scalpel." Acupotomy, performed without anesthesia, can be used to ease soft-tissue lesions and remove abnormal bony growths. However, successful use of the needle-scalpel demands an extraordinarily perceptive three-dimensional understanding of human anatomy.

At first glance, the small tool looks like a screwdriver. It has a sharp-bladed tip and a flat calabash-shaped handle. However, unlike the tool used by the handyman, this is a miniature surgical instrument used for treating various musculoskeletal problems particularly chronic, acute pain in the limb joints, muscles and soft tissues of the body.

Made of stainless steel, it combines a "needle" for probing and a "scalpel" for cutting. Logically, the designer of the instrument, Zhu

Hanzhang, calls it the needle-scalpel.

Since its invention, doctors around China have used it to perform delicate micro-surgery even on severe fatty tissue injuries, including slipped or crushed discs that threaten the patient's sciatic nerves or spinal cord.

Zhu Hanzhang, 48, who started out on his medical career as a barefoot doctor before training as a surgeon, is now president of the Great Wall Hospital specializing in needle-scalpel therapy, or acupotomy. Located in Changping, 30 kilometers north of Beijing, the hospital operates under the Academy of Traditional Chinese Medicine.

Through two decades of clinical practice, acupotomy has proved to be highly effective in the treatment of chronic injuries to soft tissues and abnormal bony growths that cause acute pain. By the end of 1991, Zhu and his trainees had treated 1.2 million patients suffering from these two types of ailments, with an unbelievable cure rate of 88.3 percent.

Acupotomy is now being used to treat at least 10,000 cases a day throughout China. It is a non-invasive style of surgery. The *acupotomist* does not open the body of the patient, as a conventional surgeon does. He performs closed surgery without breakage of the skin or bleeding.

As the combination of the needle and scalpel suggests, Dr. Zhu's use of the instrument is a manipulation between acupuncture, which uses a needle, and surgery, which uses a scalpel. Zhu describes it as being slightly closer to acupuncture than surgery. "In fact, needle-scalpel therapy has grown out of acupuncture," he says.

However, acupuncture's function is limited to stimulation. Where cutting or separating of soft tissues or bony growths is required, it is of no use. That is why Zhu added a blade onto the needle's tip.

"The idea is to carry out acupuncture therapy and surgery simultaneously — the needle-scalpel allows just that to be done."

Dr. Zhu claims that if an accurate diagnosis is made, and if the needle-scalpel is properly used, acupotomy can provide up to "100 cures in 100 cases" in treating chronic soft-tissue lesions and at least "95 cures in 100 cases" in treating overgrowths of bone. It can even work in cases otherwise diagnosed as inoperable.

Acupotomy is recognized as an operative treatment directed at an affected region without causing any damage to healthy tissues.

Manipulations can help separate abnormal adhesions and scrape away scar tissue (the excess tissue that grows when an injury heals) in or between bones, muscles, ligaments, nerves, blood vessels and aponeuroses.

Doctor Zhu estimates that he can treat approximately 130 different chronic soft-tissue lesions, some of the most-common being tennis elbow, shoulder-neck syndrome, backache and lumbar muscle strain.

In his early years, Zhu studied acupuncture and anatomy. Mastery of anatomy, he says, is a prerequisite for practicing needle-scalpel therapy successfully. "You may not see a damaged or diseased area but you have to envisage exactly what lies under the skin," he says.

In 1968, Zhu went back to his home village in Shuyang County, Jiangsu Province, after graduating from high school. It was during this period of the cultural revolution (1966-1976) that he became a rural medic, serving local farmers. At this time he also poured over a huge collection of medical classics that once belonged to his grandfather.

Separation of Adhesions

In the spring of 1974, Zhu treated his first chronic soft-tissue lesion case when he was only 25 years of age, while acting as director of the orthopedics and traumatology division of a local hospital.

The patient was Huang Jiaxiang, a carpenter in his early 40s. His right hand had been struck by an axe and it had swollen to an horrific size. Surprisingly, X-ray pictures showed no fracture or dislocation of bones. Application of poultices and ointments containing medicinal herbs did reduce the swelling, but the hand remained deformed. Only after failing to respond to physiotherapy and acupuncture in Nanjing did the carpenter approach Dr. Zhu in his local hospital.

Dr. Zhu recalls "After an initial examination, I had a notion that adhesions under the skin limited the free movement of muscles in the hand."

The doctor decided to separate the adhesions. He inserted a No.9 injection syringe into the palm of the deformed hand and plucked there for about 30 seconds before withdrawing it. "I was trying to separate the adhesions between the aponeuroses of lumbrical muscle and the palmar flexor digitorum," he says. Zhu then massaged the stiffened hand, "to stabilize and attune the hand to the separation."

Three days later the carpenter returned to the hospital with remarkable news. He could move his hand quite normally. And he felt no soreness whatsoever.

Encouraged by the results of this bloodless operation with a syringe, Zhu continued to use, with similar success, No. 9 syringes to treat chronic injuries to soft tissues. But eventually he abandoned their use in favor of a set of self-designed needles tipped with tiny blades. He called them small needle-scalpels.

Recognition

At the end of 1975, an investigation group from the public health bureau of Huaiyin City watched Dr. Zhu perform needle-scalpel therapy on soft-tissue lesions and checked-up on the recovery of 100 patients who had received the treatment.

Their findings, published in a report, attracted the attention of the Jiangsu Provincial Science and Technology Commission which decided in May 1976 to offer Zhu a grant equal to US$3,400 for further research into small needle-scalpel therapy for the clinical treatment of chronic soft-tissue lesions.

Dr. Zhu carried out his research in Shuyang County Hospital of Traditional Chinese Medicine, where he would eventually be elevated to vice-president. During this time he was often invited to practice in several Nanjing hospitals to promote his acupotomy techniques. Again he worked miracles with his small needle-scalpels by successfully treating many patients that other doctors had failed to cure. On the basis of such encouraging results, Jiangsu Provincial Health Bureau decided to grant the equivalent of US$6,000 to conduct a follow-up appraisal on 289 cases treated by Dr. Zhu in Nanjing between 1981 and 1984.

The treated cases included syndrome of the third lumbar vertebra transverse process (L_3TP Syndrome), scapulohumeral periarthritis, tennis elbow, heel spur, injury of the knee joint's medial collateral ligament and peripheral connective tissues, lumbosacral strain and tenosynovitis stenosans.

In September 1984, nine osteotraumatic experts from Nanjing's hospitals presented the results of their appraisal on Zhu's small needle-scalpel practices. Short-term follow-up results showed an effective rate of 92.7 percent. Three years later, long-term follow-up results showed an effective rate of up to 96 percent.

In the same year, Zhu set up the 100-bed Nanjing Jinling Hospital for Osteotraumatic Diseases, the first of its kind in the country devoted

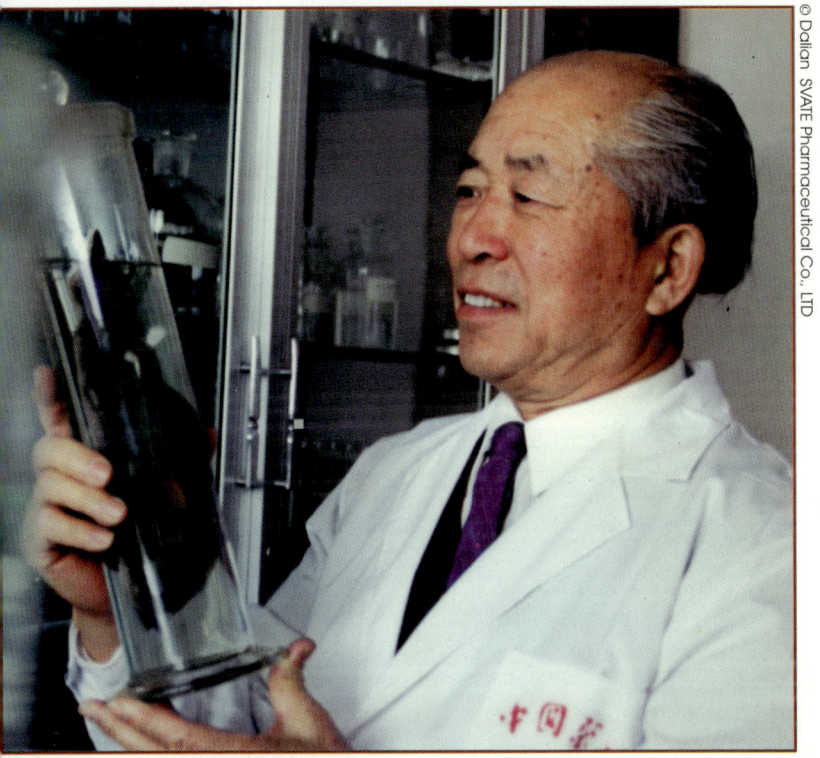

Fig.1 Hao Wenxue, the snake venom expert, scrutinizes a preparation during research to develop a new generation anti-thrombus enzyme.

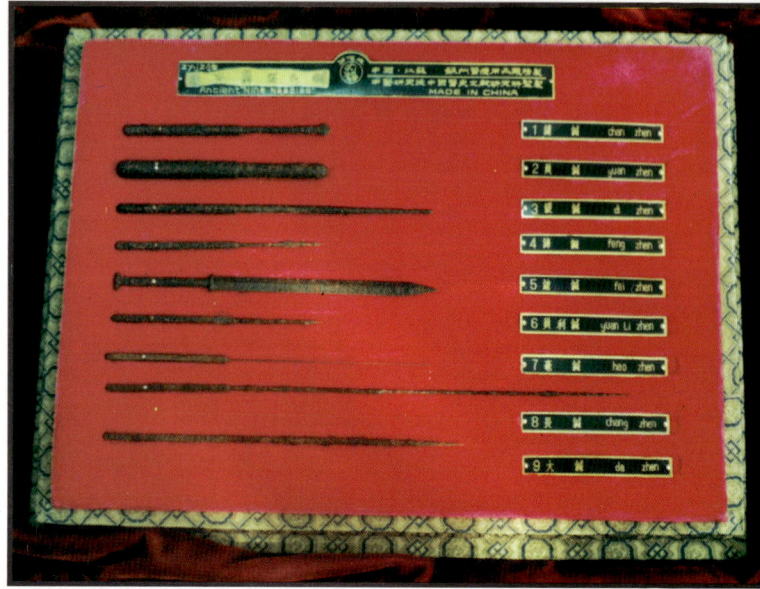

Fig.2 A replica set of the Ancient Nine Needles.

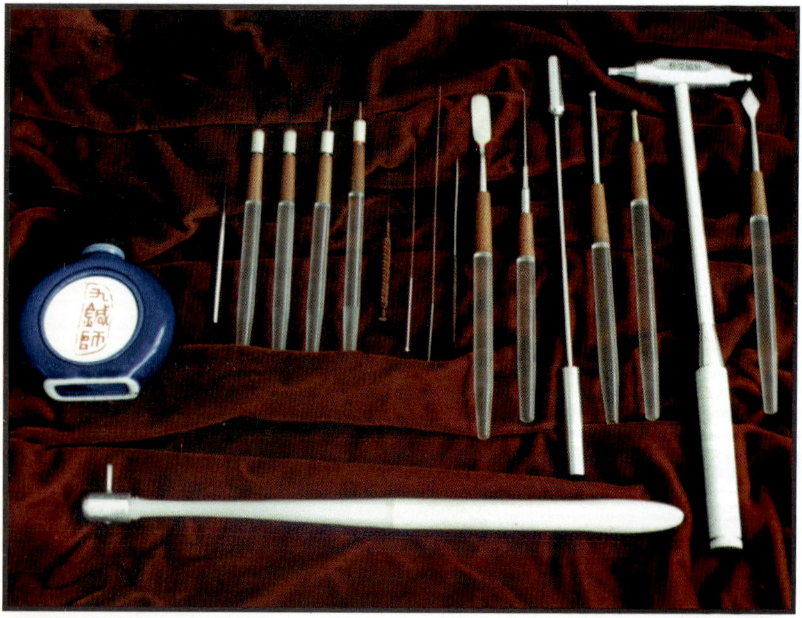

Fig.3 Revived New Nine Needles designed by Shi Huaitang (from right to left). Arrowhead Needle; Round and Plum-Blossom Magnetic Percussive-Punctator; Blunt Needles (3rd-5th); Hooked Needle; Sword-Shaped Needle; Round and Sharp Needle; Capillary Needles (8th-10th); Fire Needles (11th-15th); Three-Edged Needle; Plum Blossom Needle (horizontal).

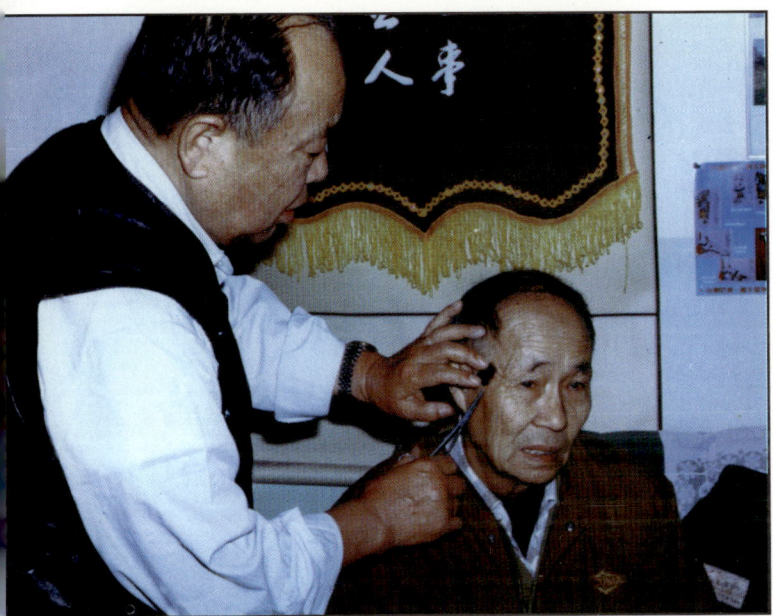

Fig.4 Shi Huaitang in the process of removing a cancerous mole (black) from the temple of patient Wang Zuoyu. A Sword-Shaped Needle with heat was used for the operation, performed in 1985.

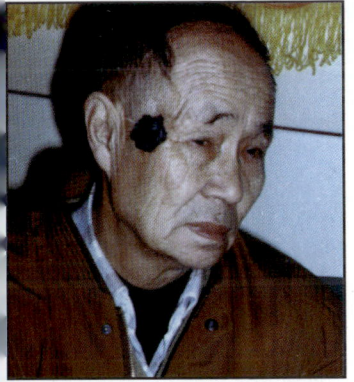

Fig.5 Wang Zuoyu before treatment.

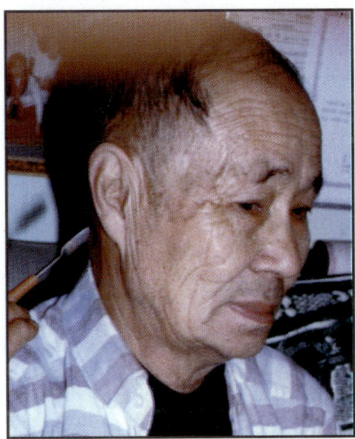

Fig.6 Wang Zuoyu after treatment.

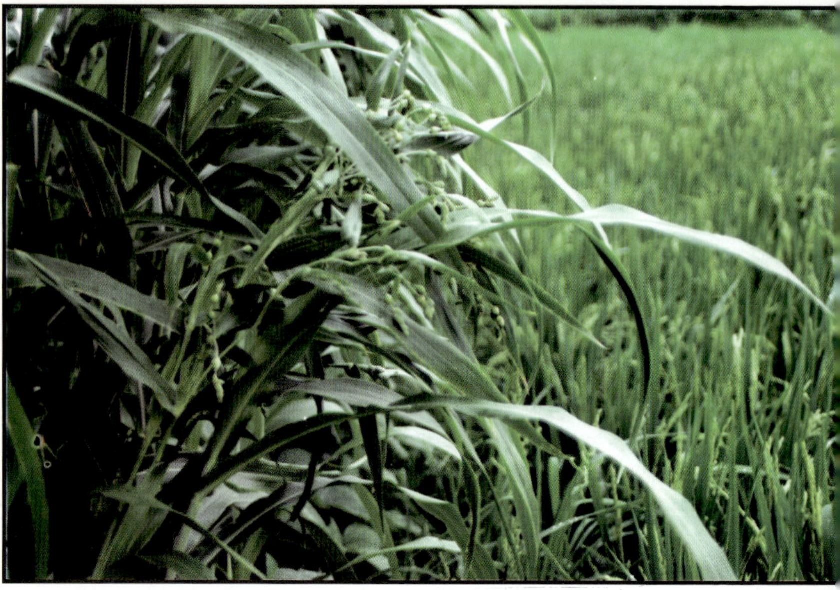

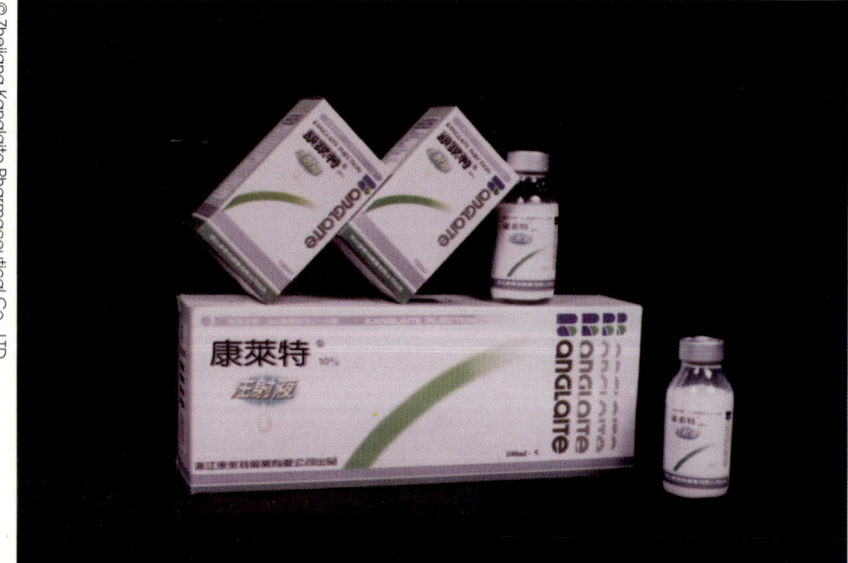

Fig.7 The grass Job's Tears, source of the sole ingredient of *Kanglaite*. The plant is indigenous to South China.

© Zhejiang Kanglaite Pharmaceutical Co., LTD

Fig.8 Packages of *Kanglaite* Injection.

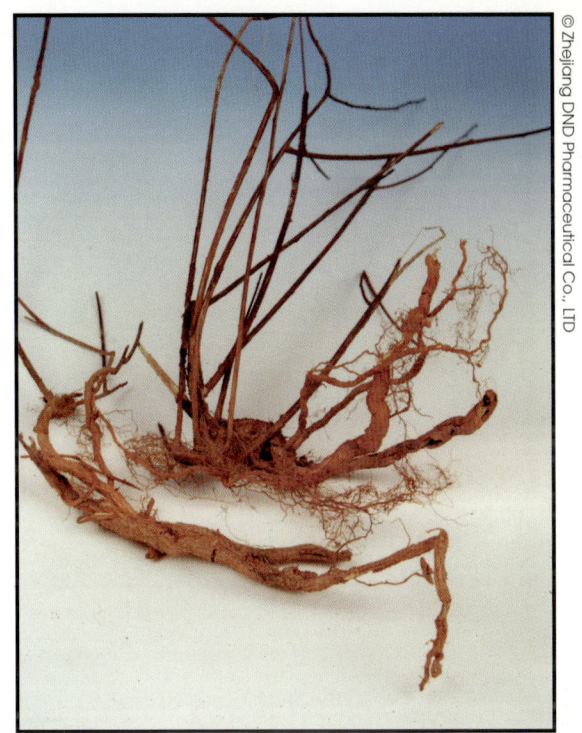

Fig.9 Dried roots and stems of *Lei Gong Teng* (*Triptergium Wilfordii*).

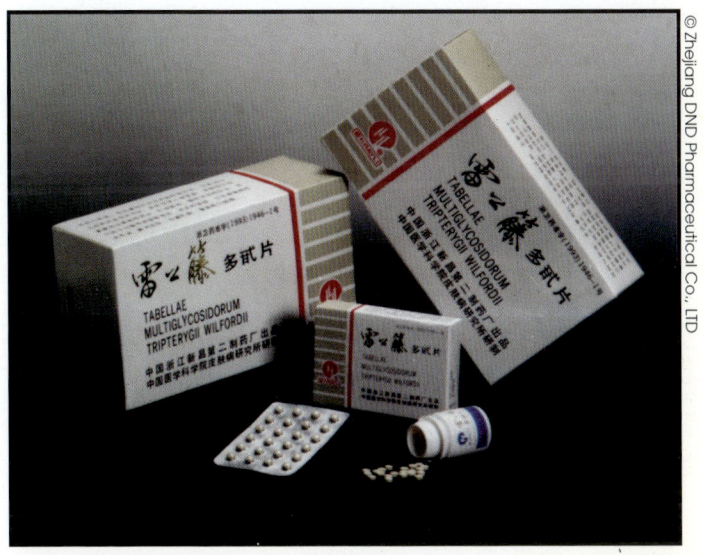

Fig.10 Packaged *Triptergium Multiglycoside*.

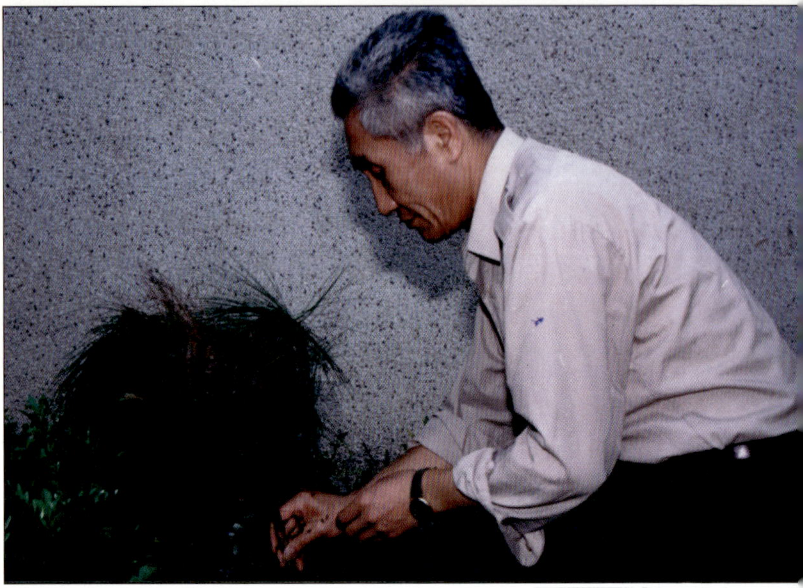

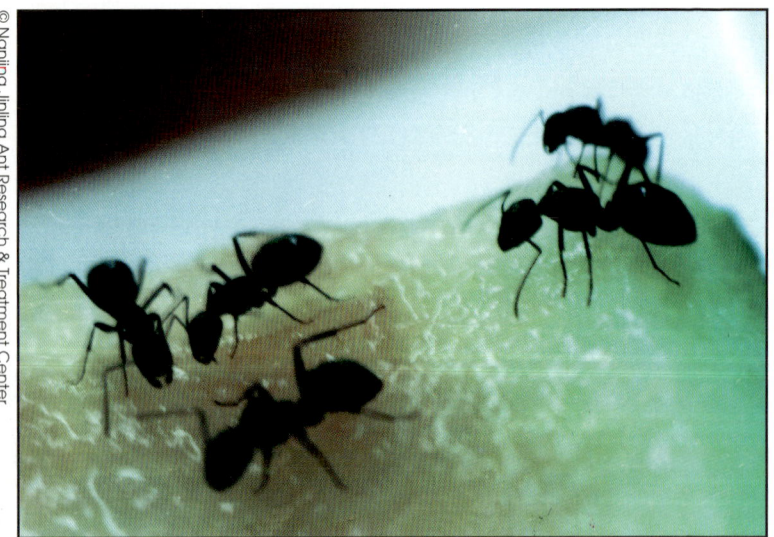

Fig.12 Wu Zhicheng looks for mountain ants at Zhenlongshan, Guangxi Zhuang Autonomous Region.

Fig.13 Black ants, first collected in 1981-82, from Tianyang County, Guangxi Zhuang Autonomous Region, and identified as *Polyrhachis Vicina Roger*.

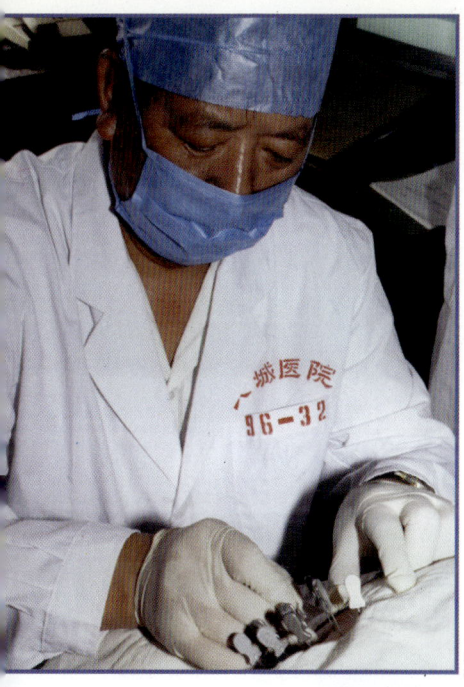

Fig.15 Zhu Hanzhang performs needle-scalpel closed surgery on Wu Xiaoyuan, an overseas Chinese from the Philippines. Wu was suffering from *ankylosing-spondylitis* hunchback.

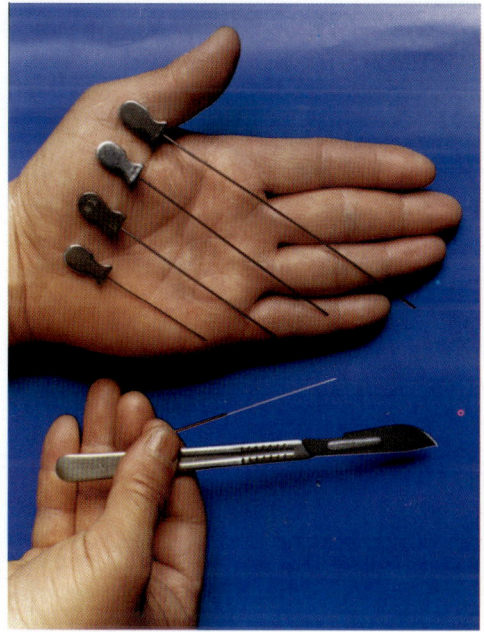

Fig.14 Small needle-scalpels (left hand), Type I Nos.1-4 (long to short), are combinations of the needle and scalpel held in the right hand.

Photo by Xue Tiejun

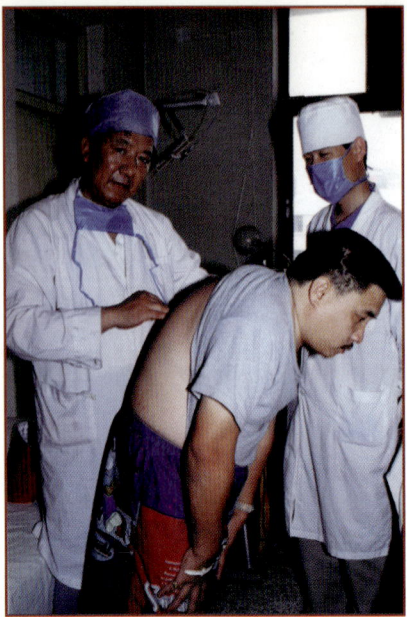

Fig.16 Wu Xiaoyuan, exhibiting chronic hunchback posture, being measured before the commencement of treatment.

Photo by Xue Tiejun

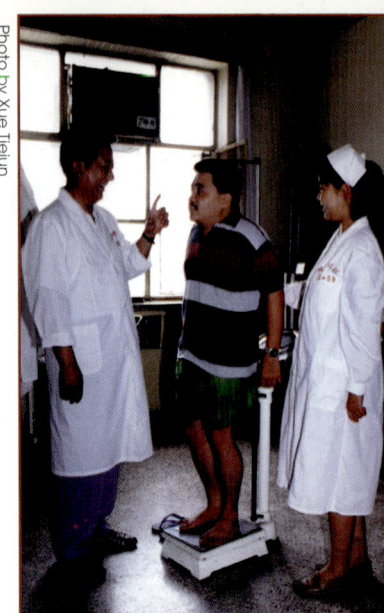

Fig.17 From May 4, 1995, 33-year-old Wu received 14 small needle-scalpel operations. After this course he was measured at 1.55m with improved posture, 11cm taller than before.

Photo by Xue Tiejun

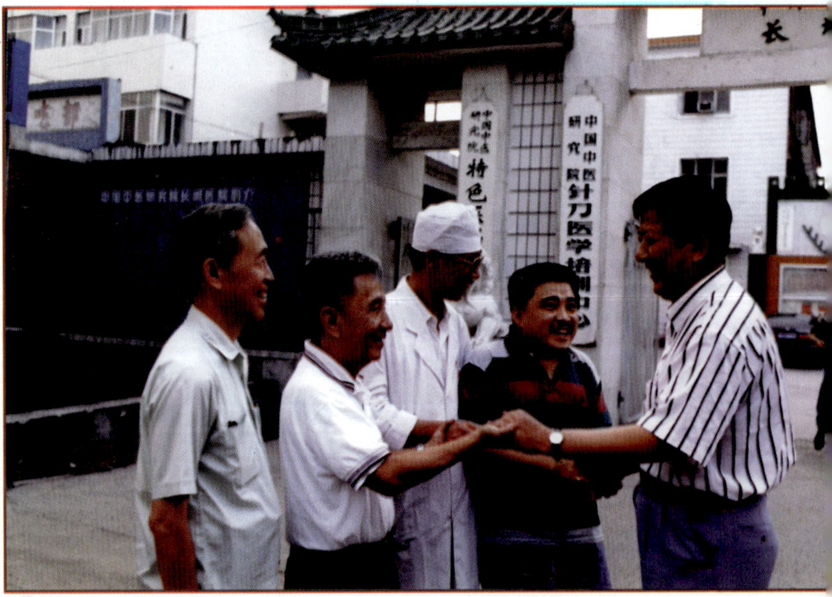

Fig.18 A delighted Wu Xiaoyuan on leaving hospital after a 59-day course of treatment.

to needle-scalpel closed surgery.

To date, Zhu has published more than 20 monographs and compiled three works to help train more acupotomists. They include: *Small Needle Scalpel Therapy*; *Zhu Hanzhang's Acupotomy: Diagnostic & Treatment Basics*; and *Lectures on Acupotomic Manipulations*. He has also translated *Knee Joints Surgery* and *Lumbago* into Chinese.

In March 1988, Zhu was awarded a patent right for his instrument — the small needle-scalpel — by the national patent office. In December of the same year acupotomy was awarded a gold medal at the 37th Brussels Eureka World Fair for Invention (research and industrial innovation) and Dr. Zhu himself won the Officer Medal.

A training program was first launched in 1987, according to Wang Xiaozhi, deputy director of the Training Center of Acupotomology under the Academy of Traditional Chinese Medicine. Up to now, 40 national and 100 local training classes have been organized, training a total of 12,000 acupotomy surgeons throughout China.

Zhu has personally trained 63 intermediate and senior acupotomy surgeons, 32 of whom now work in Zhu's Great Wall Hospital, which opened in July 1994.

Since 1990 acupotomy has aroused interest outside its native China. Surgeons trained by Zhu have been invited to lecture and open clinics in 37 countries and regions including Taiwan, Thailand, Singapore, South Korea, Japan, Australia, Russia, Germany, Brazil and South Africa. In addition, scholars from Japan and Russia have been to China to study the therapy.

Manipulation

Closed surgery is conducted under sterile conditions. The surgeon wears sterilized gloves and a gauze mask. The patient wears a sterilized drape with an opening at the appropriate part of the body under investigation.

A dye, gentian violet, is used to mark appropriate insertion points or target focuses. Generally, anesthesia is unnecessary, but a local anesthetic may be administered for closed orthopedic surgery on patients with bow-legs or knock-knees. There is no bleeding and only a slight bruise is left on the skin after treatment. This can be patched with a small piece of gauze. After three days the patient can remove it and take a shower.

Patients suffering from hepatitis, internal inflammation and hemophilia should not be treated with acupotomy. Those with open sores or ulcerations on the skin's surface at the necessary insertion points cannot receive treatment either.

Regarding rehabilitation, few patients require prescription of anti-inflammatory medicines. However, herbal medicine is recommended to promote blood circulation and prevent clotting. The same can also be used for rheumatoid arthritis cases as it helps to restore the function of affected joints.

Generally, one or two treatments are enough to cure a case, with one or two "ouch" points being found. An ouch point is a place where the patient feels pain when pressure is applied on the skin. More treatment can be given to severe cases with the interval between treatments being 5-7 days during which the practitioner can monitor the patient's response to treatment. But this depends on the individual. Some patients recover quicker than others.

Zhu holds that no part of the body is too remote to be treated by acupotomy. "It can even reach into cervical and lumbar vertebrae, internal organs and blood vessels," he says.

Biomechanics

Dr. Zhu's success is based on his broad-based understanding of both traditional Chinese and Western medicine, particularly anatomy.

In 1975, he studied human anatomy, bone-setting and massage in a Beijing hospital. He was then influenced in particular by *Biomechanics*, a medical work written by a Chinese-American professor, Feng Yunzhen.

From the mid-1970s Zhu began to observe and understand osteotraumatic diseases in the light of biomechanics. He found that biomechanical imbalance was the real cause of many stubborn osteotraumatic diseases.

Zhu maintains that imbalance of dynamic equilibrium is the root cause of chronic soft-tissue lesions. In a healthy state, the human body's torso and limbs can make free and flexible movements, a state called dynamic equilibrium balance. However, when affected and restricted by injuries, the body becomes disabled and limbs cannot perform their normal range of movements. This is known as dynamic equilibrium imbalance.

Hidden from view are the problems: adhesions, scar residues, and shrinkages, all resulting from traumatic and pathological injuries to soft tissues. These are the three major factors affecting relative free motions of soft tissues within their expected ranges.

Any smooth movement made by the human body requires the coordination, flexibility and accuracy of a host of muscle groups and auxiliary tissues. If adhesion, internal scar residues or spasmodic shrinkage have developed on, between or around the muscle groups, tissues or bone joints, the flexibility, accuracy and coordination of their movements will be affected. This results in pain when movements are attempted.

If any or a combination of the three pathological factors are solved, balance — dynamic equilibrium — can be recovered.

Tackling Bony Overgrowths

Western medicine regards the overgrowth and protuberance of bony tissue as a problem largely associated with aging.

But as Zhu sees it, abnormal bony growths are also caused by biomechanical problems resulting from an imbalance of inner stresses within the human body.

Zhu identifies three stress factors: traction, pressure and inflation. Where there is an abnormally high incidence of stress, spurs may grow either between joints or at the point where muscles and ligaments are attached to joints. The spur indicates the site of the abnormally high inner stress.

Many factors cause spurs, but the main culprits are strain, contracture and flaccidness of muscles and ligaments. Commonly, they occur between muscles and ligaments on the wrist, elbow, hip, knee and ankle joints.

A muscle fiber is much thinner than a strand of human hair. According to Western medicine, there are 100,000 muscle fibers per square centimeter in the human body. Every little movement involves their use.

When stressed excessively, muscle fibers, especially in the aged and non-sporting, over-stretch. They lack elasticity and tear. After this occurs, the human body attempts to strengthen the overstressed musculature by sending large quantities of calcium and phosphorus to the affected part, slowing down and stopping the damage by sclerosis formation and calcification and ossifying the accumulated calcium and phosphorus. This is called hyperosterosis, and although it is part of the body's self-repair mechanism, the amount of the repair may be too much, becoming excess bony growth that causes pain.

It follows that to cure a spur means the removal of the high stress point. Zhu uses small needle-scalpels to penetrate the center of pain and release the affected muscle fibers attached to the tip of the bone spur. The muscle fibers then shrink and regenerate through cell division, he says.

Once the high stress point is removed, the pain is gone and the bone spur gradually disappears. For example, calluses on the palm soon disappear when hands no longer do rough work.

Theory of Stagnation

"Stagnation causes pain — no stagnation, no pain." This is the belief of traditional Chinese medicine practitioners. In other words, where there is stagnation with regard to the flow of blood and the flow of vital *qi* (vital energy), pain occurs. Acupuncturists maintain that an ouch point — an area of pain — is a spot indicating the presence of disease. It follows they should also serve as treatment points.

Pain is the alarm bell of an injury, explains Zhu. "A patient always complains of pain when his injury is pressurized. Such points are the focuses of surgical attention."

In closed-surgery treatment of chronic soft-tissue lesions and bony overgrowths, about 60 percent of points selected for insertions with small needle-scalpels are ouch points. The rest are detected by the surgeon's understanding of anatomy.

During treatment the patient can tell the practitioner whether or not he feels discomfort. This is important information for the practitioner which he would be without in the case of performing a conventional operation with the patient under anesthesia.

When the needle-scalpel's tip touches the affected region, the patient responds visibly to the sensations of soreness and distention, a sign that the right spot has been found. The surgeon can then start the corrective surgery by manipulating his instrument.

But how can the surgeon manipulate his needle-scalpel so exactly?

That demands experience and anatomical knowledge — and maybe some 3-D vision. "In my mind I can clearly visualize the layout of the body's bones, muscles, blood vessels, nerves and soft tissues," says Zhu.

Based on years' clinical practice, Zhu created his own system of theories guiding closed surgery with the small needle-scalpel. This system consists mainly of: microscopic anatomy, stereoanatomy, dynamic anatomy, body surface location, a four-step insertion procedure, eight surgical manipulations, and specific closed surgery routes numbering 11 in all.

"I've learned different sense perceptions with the small needle-scalpel touching different tissues and organs," says Zhu.

A patient responds like an alarm bell during treatment. If the right focus is manipulated, the patient experiences dull soreness and distention. Sharp pain is felt if healthy muscles and blood vessels are touched. One feels a numbness if a nerve is touched only slightly, and if it is further pressurized the patient experiences extremely acute pain which feels like an electric shock.

To assist in the selection of the correct incision points, Zhu recommends examination of the patient's affected area by CT scanner, X-ray, Utrasonic-B and nuclear magnetic resonance, as well as standard physiological testing, such as blood testing.

Forbidden Areas

Heel, or calcaneal spurs, are relatively easy areas to treat because of the absence of crucial nerves and blood vessels in the vicinity of the problem, says Zhu. In contrast, closed surgeries along cervical vertebrae and inside the skull are the most difficult ones to tackle.

Explaining the effectiveness of his treatment, Dr. Zhu says that since 1984 he has treated more than 2,500 patients suffering from various blood clotting in the brain, and that "a marked improvement was observed in about 90 percent of them."

Xu Haiyang, 40, who suffered from a thrombosis, is one of those patients in Zhu's files. Referring to his case history, Zhu explains that nuclear magnetic resonance examination pictures showed clearly where a thrombus, four millimeters in length, blocked the patient's posterior cerebral artery. He could only walk on crutches and was unable to hold a pen in his right hand.

Treatment consisted of three closed surgical operations done at intervals. In the first operation to unblock the thrombus, Zhu inserted a needle-scalpel into the blocked section of the artery through the lower edge of the great occipital foramen and plucked the thrombus with a twisting action to break it.

"The insertion process was very slow," Zhu recalls. "I was cautious not to jerk the instrument even slightly for fear of damaging the vicinity and failing to reach the thrombus."

In follow-up treatment after examination of X-ray pictures, again with the needle-scalpel, Zhu targeted the fasciae on both sides of the third cervical vertabrae. This was intended to relax the fasciae and promote blood circulation in the locked artery they enveloped, thus allowing the broken thrombus to be washed away.

One week later Zhu addressed problems concerning the sequelae of the thrombosis: atrophied muscles and rigid joints. The closed surgical treatment took just ten minutes. The third and final treatment, one week later, to solve the remaining after-effect of the thrombosis, lasted just three minutes. Zhu aimed to restore movement in the patient's lower right leg.

Xu responded at each stage of treatment. After the first treatment he felt an improvement in his right leg strength. When concluded he left hospital and made a trip to climb the Great Wall. Without his crutches.

In most cases, Zhu says, the thrombus tends to jam at the section of the posterior cerebral artery. He claims that he has an 80 to 90 percent certainty of success at improving such cases.

However, because of the high skill required, none of Zhu's trainees dare to insert a small needle-scalpel into cerebral arteries.

Using needle-scalpels, Zhu also has made progress in treating other osteopathia, including old fractures, hunchback, deformities of trunk and limbs, knock-knees, bow-legs and bony arthritis.

Wang Xuetai, an eminent acupuncturist and former-president of the World Federation of Acupuncture and Moxibustion Societies, expressed admiration for Zhu's new approach of treating diseases.

He said: "I admire not only his theories of closed surgery, but also his new theories about the pathogenesis of diseases. In the treatment of chronic soft-tissue lesions, his closed surgery has been observed to be superior to the open surgery of Western medicine."

Acupotomology

Through two decades of research and practice, Zhu has established a new system of medical science, which he has termed *acupotomology*. It is a practice bridging the basic theories of traditional Chinese and modern Western medicines.

"I'd regard acupotomology as a 'compound' rather than a 'mixture' since its basic theories — pathogenesis, diagnosis and treatment, as well as its surgical instrument, the small needle-scalpel — are re-creations having their origin in the theories and practices of traditional Chinese medicine and modern Western medicine," says Zhu.

The theory of channels and collaterals of traditional Chinese medicine emerged more than 3,000 years ago when oriental philosophy characterized by abstract thinking was dominant. Modern Western medicine came into being during the Renaissance (14th-16th centuries), which saw the emergence of radical new schools of thought which advocated a more practical approach to understanding the world.

Even so, Zhu says, a possibility exists for these two different medical sciences to be fused into a new medical science. That is because their common ground — the human body — is studied and treated by both.

A modernized theory of channels and collaterals is a major component of Dr. Zhu's acupotomology. For centuries, the system of channels and collaterals, believed to exist in the human body by practitioners of traditional Chinese medicine, has been regarded as "the third conductive passage," independent of the nervous system and the blood circulation system.

Zhu maintains that the system of channels and collaterals is a unitary feedback system for human-body information activated by three conductive carriers — the nervous reflex system, the electro-physiological conducting system and the body-fluid conducting system.

The existence of the three conductive systems has been proven by means of modern sciences, Zhu says. The human body will be in a good state of balance if there is nothing wrong with these three conductive systems.

Channel points, also known as acupoints, are transmission stations of this feedback system on the human body. A group of such points interrelates with a particular set of tissues or organs. That is why acupuncture therapy on a specific group of channel points is effective for a specific ailment, but ineffective for others.

Zhu says: "Acupotomy is different from acupuncture therapy. Its manipulations can directly dredge the channels and collaterals, and improve micro-circulations. It can also create specific effects to help regulate physiological functions, activate sluggish nerve endings, adjust electro-physiological disorders and relieve the blocking of body fluid flow."

Dr. Zhu has just completed a huge medical tome entitled *Acupotomology*. The book covers acupotomology's basic theories, physiology and pathology, as well as diagnostics, acupotomic images, therapeutics, manipulations and nursing care.

Dr. Zhu says that it is easier for surgeons practicing Western medicine, rather than those specializing in traditional Chinese medicine, to learn acupotomy. That is because the former already have a systematic knowledge of anatomy, physiology and pathology.

Needle-scalpels are now produced solely by Beijing Huaxia Needle-Scalpel Medical Instrument Factory. Output stands at 20,000 instruments per month in three types: I, II and III.

Type I includes four needle-scalpels, each with a diameter of one millimeter: they are used on soft tissue lesions and bony growths. Type II is two millimeters in diameter: it is used for closed orthopedic surgery on bow-legs and knock-knees. Type III is three millimeters in diameter: it is used for other colsed orthopedic surgery. All three types of small needle-scalpels have the same cutting edges (at their tips) of 0.8 millimeters. The longest one is 15 centimeters while the shortest is seven centimeters.

Future plans at Changping's Great Wall Hospital include the construction of an 18-story building to add to the original one which already provides 370 beds. The number of beds will increase to 1,000 to meet the demand of patients at home and abroad.

"More sophisticated diagnostic equipment will be purchased to enable acupotomy to be widely applied in the clinical treatment of more ailments," Dr. Zhu says. "We also hope to exchange views on acupotomy with experts from the rest of the world. For centuries, traditional Chinese medicine and modern Western medicine have developed along their own widely divergent lines. There has been a lack of communication between the two medical systems because of people's different intellectual approaches and the language barrier. But today, modern technology and globalization have provided more favorable conditions for frequent communication," he says.

"Since the goal of all medicine is to effect optimum healing with minimum discomfort to patients," says Dr. Zhu, "why don't we work for a fusion of traditional Chinese medicine and modern Western medicine for achieving this ultimate aim."

FOR RELEVANT ILLUSTRATIONS, SEE Figs. 14-18.

CHAPTER 10

A PHARMACY IN A TINY BOTTLE

Yunnan Baiyao, literally meaning Yunnan White Medicine, smells like a walk through an exotic forest. That's a clue to its composition: a dozen or so herbs from the southwestern flora-abundant province of Yunnan — but exactly which herbs remains a state secret. Successfully used for more than 80 years, Yunnan Baiyao, now available in several forms, is a veritable cure all and an essential, trusty family medicine in China.

In October 1995, China's Ministry of Public Health made public the names of Chinese medicines under state protection. Only two medicines were listed in the top, most-secret category. (It is commonplace in China for inventors of herbal medicines to vigorously conceal the composition of their preparations). One of these most-secret medicines was *Yunnan Baiyao* (*YB*).

Yunnan is a province of southwest China. *Baiyao* originated there, but it is now known far beyond the borders of the mountainous region bordering Tibet, Burma, Laos and Vietnam. The reason? Its truly panacean properties and a vividly-recorded history.

The complete pharmacy in a bottle, so small that it can easily be concealed in a clenched fist, can arrest hemorrhages, heal festering wounds, activate blood circulation, disperse blood clots, eliminate inflammation and swelling, expel pus, and counteract toxins. It is especially good for *Dieda Sunshang*, or injuries from falls, fractures, bruises and strains.

Legendary Cures

Yunnan Baiyao is probably the most highly and widely respected medicine in China today. It can be found in many homes in the country. Numerous renowned cases since the early 1900s testify to the power of the white powder while millions of individuals have their own personal experiences.

One of the best known case histories occurred circa 1912, in Yunnan Province. A peasant boy named Li had his index finger chopped off while cutting grass. The boy's mother immediately fetched some white powder from the family's medicine box, washed the wound, and sprinkled it on. She optimistically connected the severed finger, then wrapped her son's hand tightly with a piece of cloth.

When the cloth was removed about 20 days later the boy's finger had knitted itself back on. He could use it quite normally. In fact the only trace of the injury was a scar.

More than 70 years later, in February 1983, Jiang Jialun, a Chinese marine biologist, fell overboard while on an Antarctic exploration voyage. He was in the freezing water for 30 minutes before being hauled out — on the brink of death. For the next two days he suffered from acute exposure, with his temperature being seven degrees Celsius below normal. He also had a persistent pain in his stomach and kept vomiting. A foreign doctor treated him to the best of his abilities, to no avail. Then Jiang remembered that he had a bottle of *YB* in his rucksack: the medicine is an essential for Chinese traveling in remote parts. Jiang took a dose by washing the white power down his throat with warm water. Shortly afterwards, his stomach ache disappeared, vomiting stopped and his body temperature began rising.

Case histories like these, spread by word of mouth, have made *Baiyao* almost legendary. But what is the medicine made from, and what is the pharmacological basis of its remarkable functions? Few doctors can tell.

Only a handful of people in China can explain *YB*'s miracle-like functions. But even if questioned they tend not to reveal any details.

By smelling *Yunnan Baiyao* one can deduce that it is a natural product. It is made from a dozen or so herbs indigenous to Yunnan, which has one of the most diverse assemblages of plants in the world due to its temperate and sub-tropical climates. One herb, *Sanqi* (*Panax Notoginseng*), is believed to be the main ingredient. It has long been acknowledged in China that *Sanqi*, also called *Tianqi*, can effectively stop bleeding, dissolve clots and promote blood circulation. *Sanqi* is used in several other Chinese medicines to induce more or less similar effects.

Applications of *YB* are extensive: a book by Yang Jucai and others published in 1995 describes in detail the effective use of the powder for more than 100 illnesses. Some applications would never have been dreamed of by its legendary inventor, Qu Huanzhang.

Unmatched Medical Skills

According to one account, Qu was born in 1880 (the sixth year of the reign of Emperor Guangxu of the Qing Dynasty) in Zhaoguan, a village in Jiangchuan County, Yunnan. When he was 12 years old, he started to learn traditional Chinese traumatology from Yuan Enlin, his sister's father-in-law. At the same time he was taught to make up prescriptions.

A personal trauma that befell Qu in the city of Gejiu in 1896 might be considered as the root of *Yunnan Baiyao*. He was hit by a severe pain in the belly that almost claimed his life. Yao Lianjun, a local herbalist of great fame, brought him round. After recovery, the impressed Qu became the herbalist's student. It is said that he inherited all the medical knowledge that the old herbalist had accumulated over a lifetime.

After Yao's death, Qu practiced medicine on his own. He visited the mountains in southern Yunnan, trying various medicinal herbs, calling on local herbalists and herb growers, and gathering well-known prescriptions.

Finally, around 1902, he formulated a prescription mainly for treating *Dieda Sunshang*, or injuries from falls, fractures, bruises and strains. It contained *Sanqi* and a few other local herbs, but *Sanqi* was the main ingredient.

Qu's medicine was used to treat soldiers wounded in wars among the many warlord factions at that time. It grew to be highly valued for its speedy, effective functions.

The story about Qu's treatment of Wu Xuexian, a local bandit, is one of the medicine's most famous tales. It happened on a certain day in the mid-1910s. Qu had a group of unexpected visitors —

supporters of Wu — who demanded that he go with them to treat their chief, who had been shot in the chest. Qu saved chieftain Wu's life in a couple of days by administering the white powder — *Yunnan Baiyao*.

From then on bandit Wu became a *Baiyao* believer. By 1918 he had become a lieutenant general under Tang Jiyao, a general of the Kuomintang army. The following year, during the Kuomintang's Northern Expedition aimed at toppling the rule of the northern warlords, Wu was shot again, this time in his right leg. Doctors treating him in Kunming, the provincial capital of Yunnan, deemed amputation to be his only chance of survival. But Wu recalled the remarkable treatment Qu had given him years before. The herbalist was found and a miracle repeated. Wu walked normally after being treated with *Yunnan Baiyao* for the second time in his life.

When the news reached Tang, he appointed Qu director of the native Yunnan Medicine Department of a well-known local hospital. General Tang also presented Qu with an honor board (a plaque on which Chinese characters were inscribed) bearing the words "Unmatched Medical Skill in Southern Yunnan."

Origin of the Name

In the early years, Qu did not give his medicine a definite name. People described it according to its appearance or its famous inventor-administrator: *Baiyao* (white medicine) or *Qu's Baiyao*. In 1916, when he was 36, Qu applied for government recognition for his medicine. It was approved and registered for public sale, with the name *Baibaodan* (one-hundred-treasure medicine).

The medicine sold so well that other pharmacists tried to produce it. To protect his product, Qu developed a tiny, red pill. Each bottle of his powdered medicine contained one such pill (it still does to this day), which was later called *Baoxianzi*, or the "safety pill." The ball distinguished the authentic medicine from fakes, and also kept the powder from deteriorating. More importantly, the pill, a stronger form of *Baiyao*, can be used for very serious problems.

In the early 1930s, Qu built and ran a drug store in Jinbi Street, Kunming. He also published a booklet entitled *Qiu Sheng Lu* (*Life-Saving Prescriptions*) to publicize his products. His annual sales volume at the time amounted to 30,000-40,000 bottles.

In July, 1937, Qu went to Chongqing, China's wartime capital, at the invitation of a high-ranking Kuomintang official, Jiao Yitang. In the name of fighting the Japanese, Jiao demanded that Qu disclose his *Baiyao* prescription so that it could be mass produced by his own pharmaceutical factory. Qu refused. He was placed under house arrest and died just a month later, supposedly of depression, aged 57.

Prescription under State Care

After Qu's death, his widow Miao Lanying and her son continued to make and sell *Baibaodan*, as it was still known, in Kunming. Not long after the founding of New China in 1949, the Ministry of Public Health sent special representatives to ask Miao to offer her husband's prescription to the state. She finally agreed in November 1955.

Since then, Qu's *Baibaodan* prescription has been under state care and kept strictly confidential. Production of the medicine was initially undertaken by the fifth workshop of Kunming Pharmaceutical Factory. The medicine was officially renamed *Baiyao*, or White Medicine.

On June 1, 1971 the fifth workshop became a factory, the Yunnan Baiyao Factory (YBF), in its own right. Qu Wanzeng, the eldest son of Qu Huanzhang, served as the factory's advisor. In its first year the plant turned out 12.97 million bottles.

Since the establishment of the YBF, staff have pressed ahead with research on the medicine.

According to Gao Chongkun, director of the Research Institute of YBF, experiments were carried out in the early years to farm the herbal constituents of *YB*. The work was successful but results showed that it took too long for farmed plants to mature to the required sizes. Besides, the natural supply of wild plants was abundant in Yunnan. Cultivation of wild herbs, therefore, was excluded from the production process.

The 1980s saw remarkable expansion of the YBF, when the government invested 14 million yuan (about US$1.68 million) to better its production facilities. New buildings for production and research were built. Among the 500 pieces of modern equipment installed in the factory were German and Japanese automated-production lines and machines for loading and packaging. This made it possible for the factory's researchers to develop new forms of *YB*.

In November 1993 the factory was transformed into *Yunnan Baiyao* Industry Co., Ltd. (YBICL).

However, there are still three small pharmaceutical factories in

Yunnan which make what is touted as the same medicine. Their products are supposedly based on the same prescription but are priced lower than YBICL's. Li Zhiguang, deputy general manager of YBICL, estimated that the combined production of the three factories in 1995 was roughly equal to that of YBICL.

Capsules, Tincture, Bands

In the past 20 years several new forms of *YB* have been developed. Some are thought even more effective than the traditional powder when treating certain conditions. YBICL has virtually no domestic rivals in these forms of the medicine.

The *YB* capsule was mass produced in 1985. The medicine is easier to administer than the powdered form. Also, accurate dosage is no longer a problem. When external application is necessary, the patient can simply pull apart the capsule and use the powder inside.

The tincture form, a mixture of the powder with alcohol, was also launched in 1985. The medicine has, for a long time, been recommended to be administered with wine: the tincture provides this convenient ready-mixed form. Early clinical practices have shown that it is especially good for treating chilblains, a common problem in China.

Yunnan Baiyao adhesive plasters, introduced in 1985, are sterile and curative patches to cover external wounds. In addition, they prolong the duration of the medicine's effectiveness and help it better penetrate the skin. The plaster is especially effective for treating injuries in which the skin is not broken.

The aerosol was developed from 1991 onwards, finally reaching consumers in early 1996. In this form, medicine and the refrigerant combine to stop bleeding and relieve pain. The aerosol is the easiest form of *YB* to use. It is reportedly very popular in the Xishuangbanna region of Yunnan Province where sugarcane-harvesting farmers are frequently cut by the razor-sharp edges of plant leaves.

All these new forms are based on the original *Yunnan Baiyao* prescription as presented to the state by the inventor's widow, Miao Lanying.

"This is still the best prescription, " said Gao Chongkun. "We attempted to change it, but none of our changes proved to be any better — so we stick with the winning formula."

The Chinese patent system began to cover traditional Chinese medicines in 1993. YBICL has recently received patent rights for its plasters and aerosols.

At present, YBICL produces mainly two series of medicines. One is called *Baiyao* series, including the various forms of *YB* and some other medicines derived from the *YB* prescription. The other is *Tianqi* series, most of which are restoratives and invigorators.

Production of the traditional bottled-powder and capsules now account for 50 percent of YBICL's total output. Production of *Gongxuening*, a capsuled medicine for women's blood diseases based on the *YB* prescription, accounts for 25 percent of total output.

In 1995, YBICL produced 10.24 million bottles or sheets of *YB* (A bubble sheet contains 16 x 0.25 gram capsules plus one red safety pill, the *Baoxianzi*). In 1996, YBICL turned out around 14 million bottles and bubble sheets.

Products of YBF carry the *Yunfeng* brand name. However, when sold abroad via foreign trade companies, they bear the *Camellia* brand name. Exports are handled by the China National Medicines and Health Products Import & Export Corporation, Yunnan Branch.

The *Yunfeng* brand is well known in China and is gaining popularity overseas. Consumers regard it as a mark of authenticity. Products of YBICL enjoy good sales in many Southeast-Asian countries and regions as well as within China. They have also found their way to Japan, Russia, the United States and Canada.

A bottle of *YB*, enough for adult dosage for 2-4 days, was sold at 1.23 yuan in 1979. Presently one needs to pay only 2.01 yuan (US$0.25) for a bottle in simple packaging and 2.97 yuan (US$0.38) for a bottle in deluxe packaging.

FOR RELEVANT ILLUSTRATIONS, SEE Figs. 19 & 20.

CHAPTER 11

THREADS SOAKED IN MYSTERY

Rising coils of scented smoke intensify the aura of mystery surrounding the curative effects of the hot hemp thread as it is pressed onto a patient's skin. The treatment, targeting acupuncture points, was for centuries only practiced within the confines of a single ethnic Zhuang family living deep in the hills of south China's Guangxi region. Long Yuqian decided to popularize the benefits of the smoldering alcohol- and musk-soaked thread, and perfect its use to cure hosts of health problems ranging from infertility to eczema.

In the West, thread is used to stitch up gaping wounds and repair the incisions through which surgery has been performed. In China thread is used in the same way, but in Guangxi Zhuang Autonomous Region it is used as a medicine itself.

The thread in question is 30cm long and 1mm in diameter. It is said to effectively treat more than 100 diseases.

Mrs. Huang had been infertile for six years. She tried all available treatments in Hong Kong, but still she could not conceive. When in 1987 she traveled to Guilin, a scenic city in Guangxi, as a tourist, she happened to hear about the thread from local people and decided to have a try.

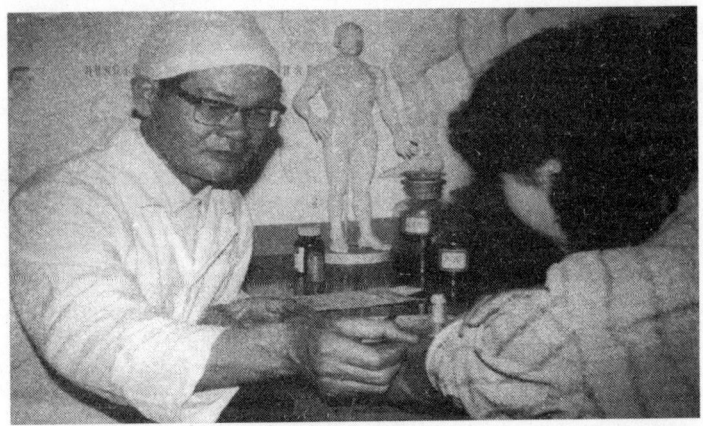

Huang Jinming applies a smoldering medicated thread to the acupoint of a patient's forearm.

She spent 24 days in the city receiving treatment in a clinic operated by Long Yuqian, master of this therapy. Afterwards, her menstrual cycle returned to normal, her womb position corrected and she was declared "recovered."

In April 1990, she mailed a picture of her baby girl to Long, with a letter of thanks. "I might never have had a baby of my own without your treatment," she said in her letter. "My daughter and I will never forget what you've brought to us."

What cured Mrs. Huang of her infertility was just a piece of thread. But not an ordinary one. Made from hemp fibers, it is immersed in alcohol, musk and 11 other herbal medicines for 48 hours before being applied on the patient's body acupuncture points.

The treatment process is simple. First, one end of the medicated thread is ignited, then the flame is extinguished after a few seconds. The smoldering end is applied to an acupoint. Then the practitioner presses his thumb on the point with a downward twisting force.

This therapy is an heirloom of the Long family who have resided in Liuzhou, Guangxi, for generations. The family is Zhuang, an ethnic minority people inhabiting South China.

Long Yuqian, 65, learned the process of treatment and healing techniques at an early age from his father and grandmother. He is the latest in his family to carry on the practice.

Dr. Long claims the thread therapy can treat or cure more than 100 diseases, including tuberculosis, infertility, neurological and kidney diseases, diarrhea, acute strains and eczema (a red swollen condition of the skin).

Since 1974, he has treated more than 100,000 patients, of whom 80 percent have improved their conditions according to his case records.

Standard Principles

The thread treatment follows the same principles as acupuncture and moxibustion, both common therapies of traditional Chinese medicine. According to the theory, a disease is caused by an imbalance of the vital *qi* (internal energy of the body) that flows along a system of channels believed to exist in the human body, as well as an imbalance of blood flow. Healing is achieved by stimulating selected points distributed on or along the main and collateral channels. In other words, treatment aims to balance and regulate the *qi* and blood.

The difference between the two therapies is that, in acupuncture, the balance of *qi* and blood is achieved by inserting and rotating long needles into the points, while the thread therapy achieves the result by giving warm, medicated stimulation to the points.

Of the body's total acupoints, 362 are used in the thread therapy, according to Long. The therapy shares most of the points with acupuncture. "At some shared points, the thread therapy and acupuncture serve different purposes, and there are some points used in thread therapy only," he says.

Three types of medicated thread are used, each 30cm long. Thread No.1, 1mm in diameter, is generally used in winter and applied to acupoints where the skin is relatively thick. Thread No.2, 0.7mm in diameter, is the most commonly used. Thread No.3, 0.25mm in diameter, is made for children and applied to acupoints where the skin is relatively thin.

Generally, one course of treatment lasts 15 days. Every day the patient receives one stimulation with the smoldering, medicated thread. "Sometimes I twist two types of thread together to treat chronic and stubborn diseases," Long says. The patient is charged three to five yuan (less than one US dollar) each time.

In serious cases, the thread therapy is accompanied by oral doses of herbal and Western medicines to accelerate improvement.

Like other practitioners of traditional Chinese medicine, Long stresses that diagnosis and treatment should be based on an analysis of symptoms, the location of the illness and the patient's physical condition. In most cases, he makes a final diagnosis with the aid of diagnostic methods used in modern Western medicine.

The burnt thread should be kept away from the eyes. Pregnant women should avoid the treatment since the thread contains musk, which practitioners of Chinese medicine believe may cause miscarriages.

"The advantage of this therapy is that it needs no equipment other than a piece of thread and a lamp, and it doesn't induce any side effects," Long says.

Patients say there is no pain. One female patient says: "When Dr. Long applies the thread to selected points, he gives a gentle press with his thumb and I only feel a slight twinge. Only a black smear is left on the skin, but it can be wiped clean."

Long's family has kept thread making and the process of treatment a secret for several generations. In 1976, Long Yuqian started to train some apprentices in administration of the therapy.

"There were so many people coming to my clinic that I couldn't treat all of them," he says. "So I decided to train others in the therapy."

Since nothing had ever been written down about the thread therapy in Long's family, Long Yuqian had to give detailed instructions with accompanying demonstrations when he trained apprentices. The training courses were neither systematic nor regular and, for a course which lasted for about 10-15 days, he could only take on a few apprentices.

To popularize the thread therapy, Huang Jinming, a professor with the Guangxi College of Traditional Chinese Medicine in Nanning, the regional capital, who was one of Long's trainees, decided to write a book.

Huang, who is also director of the Research Institute of Zhuang Medicine at his college, opened a clinic in 1985 and invited Long Yuqian to provide treatment there.

While learning every detail of the thread therapy from Long Yuqian, Huang and ten of his colleagues formed a group to carry out research in an attempt to systemize and standardize the treatment.

Treatment Standards

Between 1983 and 1992, the group completed the technical standardization of the therapy covering its name, cure mechanism, operational method and approved method of choosing acupoints.

To study the efficacy of the therapy, the group also conducted clinical research on four different types of diseases.

One type was hemorrhagic conjunctivitis, an eye disease. Of the 125 cases treated with thread therapy alone, 104 were cured, 16 improved, while five patients showed no sign of improvement. It was effective to some degree in 96 percent of cases.

Compared with the conventional treatment of using moroxydine drops in the Ophthalmology Research Institute in Henan Province, says Huang Jinming, the thread therapy proved more effective.

Huang's clinical researchers found that the thread therapy has an effective rate of 84.5 percent for children's primary enuresis, or incontinence, 86.8 percent for dysmenorrhea (painful menstruation), and 95 percent for paralysis.

"This therapy is most effective in treating such diseases as hemicrania (pain in one side of the head), gastralgia (pain in the stomach), painful menstruation, paralysis, diarrhea, children's incontinence and epilepsy," says 58-year-old Professor Huang. He stresses that the therapy has no effects on cancer and some blood-related diseases.

The group's research findings passed an appraisal by the Public Health Bureau of Guangxi Zhuang Autonomous Region in 1992. They have been compiled into two books in 1986 and 1990. Fifty thousand copies have been sold.

Adopted Practice

Huang and his group have also run 30 training classes enrolling a total of 5,000 trainees from all over the country. Thread therapy has been put on the curriculum of the Guangxi College of Traditional Chinese Medicine.

Huang has also introduced his therapy to foreign practitioners, including some in the United States and Australia. "Today, thread therapy is practiced in 260 medical organizations throughout China," Huang says.

Though all trainees know how to administer the therapy, prescription for the liquid medicine in which the thread is soaked remains a secret to them. It is known only to Long Yuqian and Huang Jinming.

"We have applied a patent right for the prescription and have got permission to produce the thread commercially," Huang says. "We hope the magic thread can be mass produced one day."

FOR RELEVANT ILLUSTRATION, SEE Fig. 21.

CHAPTER 12

MAKING LIFE LIVEABLE WITH AIDS

There is no cure for AIDS yet. To date, a handful of Western medicines have been marketed to delay the onset of full-blown AIDS, but they are prohibitively expensive, especially for sufferers in the Third World, notably Africa, where the disease has reached plague-like proportions. Aike, a Chinese herbal preparation, is an affordable herbal hope for all HIV positives, at one-tenth of the cost of Western drugs, and without side effects.

AIDS, transmitted mainly through sexual contact, is a recently-manifested scourge which has spread around the world. It looks as if it will be one of the main killers in the next century. There is no cure at the present time for those infected with the human immunodeficiency virus (HIV) which destroys the body's ability to withstand a host of diseases.

Doctors and researchers of traditional Chinese medicine have joined the global effort to combat AIDS. After years of research and clinical work, they have come up with a herbal decoction that has been proved effective in alleviating symptoms, improving the body's immune system, and helping patients live longer and healthier lives. It is not a cure for AIDS, but tests have shown it to be a better performer than medicines developed in the West.

Commercially, the medicine is known as *Aike* Decoction (*Aike* literally means "anti-AIDS" in Chinese). It has been developed by the China Academy of Traditional Chinese Medicine (CATCM) and produced by the Svate Pharmaceutical Co. based in Dalian, a port city in northeast China.

Researchers say the medicine is most effective for AIDS patients in the early and middle stages of HIV infection, namely for AC and ARC patients, who are largely free of symptoms.

Aike is being assessed by the Ministry of Public Health and is expected to gain approval soon. The medicine will then be marketed in China and abroad.

The medicine comes in powdered form. It is packaged in sachets and taken orally after being dissolved in boiled water. Each sachet contains 10 grams of powder. Patients take the medicine twice a day, one sachet at a time.

Aike powder consists of eight varieties of herbal medicine with two herbs — *Astragalus Memranaceus* and *Viola Yedoensis* — as its main ingredients. Most of the components function to annihilate the virus and fortify the immune system.

Over the years, *Aike* has gone through rigorous clinical testing, including experimentation on animals and cell cultivation. The work shows that the herbal medicine has an efficacy rate of 51.92 percent. Most noteworthy is one case where a patient's HIV blood serum antibody turned negative after a three-month course of taking *Aike*, something unheard of since the virus was identified in 1981.

The World Health Organization (WHO) estimated in 1995 that 20 million HIV carriers existed worldwide. Worse still, more than 6,000 people contract the virus each day. Although the global fight against AIDS is a joint effort by a tremendous number of top scientists, immunologists and pharmacists funded by vast sums of money, neither a vaccine to prevent HIV infection nor a cure is in sight.

"Traditional Chinese medicine should be able to offer a way to combat AIDS since we believe AIDS largely results from the poor functions of internal organs," said CATCM Professor Wang Mianzhi, 64, who is also vice-president of the All-China Society of Traditional Chinese Medicine. "The Chinese theory is based on a comprehensive diagnosis of the body as a whole instead of approaching each part of it separately. The Chinese way to good health focuses on reinforcing the body's resistance to a disease and enhancing the function of its immune system," Wang explained.

Dual Aims

Prof. Lu Weibo, director of the AIDS Study Department under CATCM, said traditional Chinese medicine has a central tenet: *Quxie Fuzheng*, which literally means "to remove the source of evil and enhance the natural functions of the body."

"A dose or therapy aims to achieve the two functions simultaneously," he said. "For AIDS cases, we have tried to develop a medicine that can remove the HIV virus, the source of evil, and fortify the human immune system at the same time."

"This is different from Western medicine which generally pays attention only to relieving the symptoms of a disease," he explained.

Chinese herbal medicines, coming from natural plants and animals, induce almost no side effects, and some of its ingredients are also nourishing to the body, he said.

AIDS medicine widely used in the world today — *AZT*, *ddI*, *ddC* and a promising new class of drugs called protease inhibitors — are not ideal because of their serious and sometimes fatal side effects and prohibitively high costs, says Prof. Lu.

Prof. Hao Wenxue, chairman of the board of Svate Pharmaceutical Co., which makes the *Aike* decoction, shares Prof. Lu's view. He said: "The cost of *AZT* for a year's treatment is around US$2,000; besides, the medicine hinders the marrow from blood reproduction. And using a protease inhibitor for the same time might cost the patient as much as US$6,000."

"The *Aike* decoction, however, costs one-tenth of *AZT*, and it induces no side effects whatsoever."

Prof. Lu of CATCM's AIDS Research Department maintains that a combination therapy of *AZT* and *Aike* may constitute a good treatment for AIDS since *AZT*'s serious side effects can be eased by *Aike*, an effective immuno-regulator. A combination therapy can combat the immunity saboteur more efficiently, he said.

"In my view, this traditional Chinese medicine is superior to any Western medicine developed so far for dealing with AIDS," he said.

Tanzanian Experience

The WHO estimates that by 2000 the number of HIV carriers worldwide will reach 30-40 million, with 90 percent of them being found in developing countries. Africa is currently the most seriously affected continent. In Tanzania, for example, one million people were reportedly infected with the HIV virus by the end of 1995.

In 1987, at the invitation of the Tanzanian government, China and Tanzania started to cooperate in AIDS research with traditional Chinese medicine. Teams of Chinese experts have been visiting the African country in the course of their work since 1988.

Performance of the *Aike* medicine was recorded over a one-year period between August 1992 and July 1993, when a fourth team of Chinese experts worked with their counterparts in Muhimbili Medical Center, Dar es Salaam, the capital of Tanzania.

The record shows that *Aike* had an effective rate of 51.92 percent, slightly lower than *Glyke*, a Chinese herbal tablet used by the second and third teams of Chinese experts in Tanzania which had an effective performance rate of 59.62 percent.

Among the 340 patients treated with the two Chinese herbal medicines between April 1989 and August 1993, the blood serum antibody count in eight of them showed signs of a reversion from positive to negative.

Most strikingly, one patient's HIV serum antibody count turned negative after taking *Aike* for three months. The patient, B.M., 48, was tested HIV-positive after her sexual partner had died of AIDS. Before treatment, she lost eight kilograms and suffered from diarrhea and fever. Post-treatment tests showed that the HIV virus was no longer present in her blood serum, but genes of the virus still existed in her lymph cell nuclei. Basically, all AIDS-related symptoms were gone.

"It is the *Aike* decoction that has made her a long-term non-progressor," said Prof. Lu Weibo, who was also head of the fourth team of Chinese experts.

Aike was used to treat a total of 52 patients in Tanzania. During treatment, the gains and losses of their weights ranged within two kilograms. Symptoms such as fatigue, fever, cough, diarrhea, anorexia, lymphadenopathy and skin rash caused by HIV infection were alleviated by varying degrees. No serious side effects were recorded.

"*Aike* and *Glyke* were the two most effective among a dozen Chinese herbal prescriptions used on a trial basis in Tanzania. *Aike* is more persuasive in terms of efficacy and closer to international medical standards thanks to going through extensive testing on animals," Prof. Lu said.

Animal Experiments

The testing of *Aike* on animals, a key research project in China's Eighth Five-Year Plan period (1991-95), lasted five years. Research was divided into three parts: the external anti-viral experiment, the internal anti-viral experiment on small animals, and the SIV model experiment covering aetiological, immunological and pathological tests.

In the external anti-viral experiment, *Aike* was used to interact with HIV-RT, a key enzyme that the AIDS virus needs to replicate itself. Results show that *Aike* can block HIV duplication.

In the internal antiviral experiment of small animals, mice suffering from immuno-deficiency were given *Aike*. Results showed an improvement in the weakened immunity functions of the mice.

The SIV model test, developed in 1989 by WHO, is the linchpin of the whole animal experiment, according to Prof. Guan Chongfen, director of the Immunology Department of CATCM. "It is sophisticated, widely used and more persuasive since the SIVmac-infected monkeys show all the symptoms that human beings have," she said.

"We selected 12 infected monkeys — six were treated with *Aike*, three with *AZT* and three with ordinary saline water."

"The treatment lasted four months. We are elated to find that *Aike* was more effective than *AZT* in improving the monkeys' immunity functions."

Another exciting discovery was found through microscopic examination of cross-sections of these monkeys' lymph nodes. "Activation around the infected lymph nodes after treatment with *Aike* can be clearly observed, a sign that the lymph nodes were improving their function; whereas lymph nodes treated with *AZT* were observed to wither, a sign that their destruction by the virus continued," Guan said.

The result is further confirmed by laser micrography. Pictures show that the lymphocytic nucleus, after being treated with *Aike*, are under repair from a state of near disintegration before treatment, she said.

"*Aike* is effective — clinically, immunologically and serologically," she said.

Marketability

Prof. Hao Wenxue's Svate Pharmaceutical Co. purchased the

prescription for *Aike* in 1993 at a cost of two million yuan (about US$240,000). The company has since spent an additional 1.5 million yuan (US$180,000) on animal experiments involving the herbal medicine.

"The price is really very high," Hao said. "Why did I pay so much for the prescription? Because I believe it is a good medicine for AIDS patients."

Prof. Hao, who is also an eminent researcher on snake venom and the inventor of a successful medicine based on it, has no regrets about his expensive purchase.

He said: "*Aike* decoction is competitive for being both effective and economical, and most importantly, it doesn't induce side effects. Sources of its ingredients are so abundant in China that there is no problem in meeting market demand for the medicine."

"Should China face an AIDS onslaught, Chinese herbal medicine would be the best choice for Chinese patients. And traditional Chinese medicine has a high reputation in many countries, especially in Southeast Asia."

"I'm going to have this herbal medicine collar a quarter of the world market for AIDS drugs — I believe I'll make it."

Treating AIDS with herbal medicine remains a key research project in China's current Ninth Five-Year Plan period (1996-2000), according to Prof. Lu Weibo. "There are many other prescriptions that show promise in treating AIDS," he said. "We need to continue our exploration."

Quite coincidentally, Lu, Guan and Hao, the three professors directly involved in the development and manufacture of *Aike*, used to study and practice Western medicine but have all turned to traditional Chinese medicine in an attempt to combine the two for better results.

Aike may be a purely Chinese herbal medicine, but Western medical science has been extensively used for tests and analyses. With their rich experience in both Western and Chinese schools of medicine, the professors are among the most qualified to explore for an AIDS cure, using a combination of the two medical disciplines.

FOR RELEVANT ILLUSTRATIONS, SEE Figs. 22 & 23.

CHAPTER 13

EASING COLD TURKEY TRAUMAS

Authorities in southwest China's Yunnan, a province bordering Burma and the Golden Triangle which is notorious for drug trafficking and abuse, are fighting a heroin war. In their weaponry is a herbal capsule that lessens the agony of addicts' withdrawal, making their escape from the hopeless cycle of drug abuse less hell-like than ever before.

Wang Lan used to be a respectable bank accountant, but her career fell apart, as did her life, under the addiction of drugs. Since her early twenties she has been trapped in a cycle of drug dependency despite being treated in clinics on six occasions.

The woman lives in Kunming, the provincial capital of Yunnan. But with drug addiction wrecking her hopeful, young life, she really doesn't "live" any more. She just exists between fixes.

And what's even sadder is that addicts just like Wang Lan are not rarities in Kunming. The southwestern Chinese city is a blackspot for drug addiction and the Public Security Bureau (Chinese police) there knows it. They are fighting on the front line in the country's drug war.

But while they may well use arms to combat the traffickers, they have a new medicine to help the addicts. It's called *626*, after that day in June 1996 designated by the United Nations to promote awareness on the evils of drug addiction.

Wang is now a patient at the Kunming Compulsory Treatment Center for Drug Addicts. She's off heroin and on 626. It is helping her to really live again.

"Of all the medicines I've tried, the 626 capsule is the best," she says. "It's not as hard to take as many other medicines, and it doesn't make you suffer." Many of the center's other 600 compulsory and 100 voluntary patients agree.

Hell

One of the nightmares of trying to escape from drug addiction is excruciating physical and mental torment caused by withdrawal. The trauma can drive some addicts to simply an acceptance that they will be addicts forever. Others regard suicide as the only way out.

Wang says withdrawal feels like "having pains all over the body; bones itching from inside as though ants are creeping within — you don't know where to scratch, and you wish you could have your arms and legs cut off."

She says that after taking 626 capsules such symptoms are less traumatic and subside after several days. The capsule is a herbal proprietary medicine developed by the Kunming center, which is now administered by Kunming's Public Security Bureau.

A study of 1,000 addicts treated at the center with the medication shows that the capsule brings measurable relief between just five and 20 minutes after initial administration. Five to seven days of further treatment had patients in the study reporting "freedom from physical torture." Two to seven days' more treatment saw many more signs of successful withdrawal being brought about. The overall efficacy rate of the 626 capsules is 98.9 percent.

While providing rapid relief from suffering, the capsule induces none of the side effects which are commonly experienced by the taking of conventional medicines. Chronic lethargy, causing patients to sleep day and night, coupled with extreme weakness in the limbs, are common side effects. Another is memory loss. But perhaps the worst thing is that addicts become dependent on the medications which themselves are actually designed to assist in withdrawal.

An example is methadone, a chemical compound widely used by withdrawing addicts for its strong pain-killing property. While it is largely successful in gradually reducing dependence on drugs, it can in itself become indispensable to a patient. Many former heroin addicts are currently methadone addicts.

Doses of the 626 are gradually reduced during a course of treatment, which normally takes 12 days. On the first day, a patient is given three doses, each of eight capsules. Dosage is gradually reduced over the next 11 days, with only three capsules being administered on the final three days. Thus a total of 126 capsules is usually enough to treat an addict. Some patients are free of physical addiction after only eight days.

The capsule costs one-third of the price of methadone, according to a research report produced by the center.

"In addition, most patients lead a fairly normal life while taking 626," says Pan Changzhong, deputy director and physician-in-charge. He was a leading researcher in the task force which prepared the capsules.

Shen Jie, chief of the center's medical section and another leading member of the research group, says the formulation of 626 capsules is based on the principles of traditional Chinese medicine in terms of tranquilizing and calming the mind and clearing away hot and toxic substances.

Abstinence Syndrome

Through close study of the abstinence syndrome, also known as withdrawal syndrome, which is related to conventional anti-addiction medicines, Shen and his colleagues found that once the medicine on which a patient was dependent was withdrawn, active levels of body substances, such as enkephalins, dwindled dramatically. This led to both increases and decreases in the secretion of the body's series of neuro-transmitters. It is at this point that patients suffer the extreme neural, mental and digestive disorders associated with the traumas of withdrawal, often called cold turkey.

The 626 capsule comprises more than 20 medicinal herbs, including *Xueteng* (scarlet vine), *Xiaoheiyao* (small black medicine), and *Sanwu* (three blacks). Shen says about 80 percent of the herbs are indigenous and unique to Yunnan, and that quite a few of them are not even recorded in standard herbal catalogs.

Herbs in 626 activate the body's opiate receptors and serve to purge pathogenic factors, check the upward adverse flow of refined nutritive substances in internal organs, calm the mind and reinforce the functions of the spleen and stomach.

Ingredients also comprise tiny amounts of crude opium and morphine, with a combined total of no more than 5.6 milligrams per gram, Shen says. He emphasizes that such amounts cannot cause dependence, as can methadone and some opiate tinctures used in substitution therapy. Observance of more than 10,000 users of the *626* has revealed no cases of dependence development.

Drug abuse once again reared its ugly head in Yunnan during the 1980s when China's reform policy opened land border crossings between the province and its southwestern neighbors of Burma, Laos and Vietnam. Straggling the notorious Golden Triangle, southeast Asia's main center of drug production, has made Yunnan a front door to China for smugglers. They dodge detection at customs checkpoints or avoid them altogether by transporting their contraband along remote mountain and jungle tracks.

Yunnan led all Chinese provinces in the major campaign against drugs in the late 1980s, and the Kunming center was established in August, 1989 — the first of its kind in the country.

In those early days, Pan recalls, the staff were frustrated by the lack of a suitable medication to give addicts relief from withdrawal. They tried the many internationally- and domestically-used therapies and medicines, only to find them either ineffective, or effective but too costly.

He says: "As none of the established medicines were deemed desirable, we decided to develop an effective prescription based on traditional Chinese medicine, taking advantage of the rich plant resources of Yunnan. The province is known as a natural botanical kingdom."

The quest was launched in February, 1991. Pan, Shen and Zhang Zhidao, a doctor invited from the Chuxiong Hospital of Traditional Chinese Medicine, and colleagues studied numerous addiction-relieving formulas, either recorded in ancient medical books or handed down as folk prescriptions. "We even found the prescription used by Lin Zexu to cure opium addicts about 155 years ago," says Shen.

In 1839, Lin Zexu, in his capacity as Imperial Commissioner of the Qing Dynasty (1644-1911), ordered the burning of some 20,000 cases of smuggled opium confiscated from the British East-India Company, on Humen beach in Guangdong Province. This action was probably the earliest public demonstration of China's determination to stop illegal trafficking and stem drug abuse.

Members of the Kunming research group regard themselves as

successors to Lin Zexu in the campaign against drugs by developing the most effective addiction-relieving medicine to date. Having been tried in numerous compositions and subjected to thousands of clinical tests, the formula for the 626 capsule was finally settled upon in 1994.

An appraisal panel of 11 experts representing the province's top medical and pharmaceutical authorities reviewed the capsule's performance at the end of 1994. They unanimously agreed that it was an effective, addiction-breaking medication, and that its composition was well-founded, rigorously developed and, in the vast majority of cases, capable of producing desirable results. The panel predicted that the new product would play an important role in the global fight against drug abuse.

Experiments

In 1995, a group of scientists led by Professor Jiang Jiaxiong, a well-known pharmacologist of the Kunming Medical College, conducted a series of experiments on the effects of the 626 at the Yunnan Key Laboratory on Pharmacology and Toxicology of Natural Drugs.

One of the experiments compared the performances of the 626 capsule with methadone — the latter considered by many as the most effective cure for drug addicts — on different groups of heroin-dependent monkeys. The results showed the capsule had a remarkable withdrawal-easing effect comparable to that of methadone.

A very small proportion of users may feel thirsty or suffer from insomnia. These manifestations, however, cannot be compared with the physical torment resulting from taking other medicines, says Shen, who emphasizes that difficulty in sleeping is not a side effect of the 626 capsule. "Heroin is the real culprit because insomnia is part of the abstinence syndrome," he says. "The fact that some users still have sleeping problems indicates that the capsule has not yet taken full effect on those drug addicts. Some users feel sleepy. This is the very effect we expect of the capsule."

The doctor concedes that the 626 has "minimal" side effects. "We have used it in 10,000 cases now, and have observed no instances of danger in any form."

Home Therapy

Addicts can take the 626 capsules at home, but Shen warns that correct dosages must be strictly followed. He advises patients to take the capsules under supervision from family members.

A package of 120 capsules, enough for a 10-day course of treatment, costs 500 yuan (US$60) — about one-third of the cost of methadone.

The *626* capsule is targeted mainly at heroin addicts, the most commonly-used drug in Yunnan. But it has also been given to a limited number of opium, cocaine and marijuana addicts, with similarly impressive results.

So far the *626* capsule has mainly been used in drug addiction treatment centers attached to public security bureaux throughout Yunnan. Its production, controlled by the Kunming center, is in batches of 10,000 packages manufactured on a sporadic basis.

The center was given the go-ahead by the provincial Public Health Department and the Pharmaceutical Administration to establish its own Kunming Kangqi Pharmaceutical Plant, which went into operation in early 1997.

The plant is located within the center's walled compound. With an investment of 1.2 million yuan (US$150,000), it is equipped with modern pharmaceutical manufacturing facilities. First-year production totaled 30,000 small packages. "This is adequate to meet the demand in Yunnan Province," says center director Zhang Yuzu.

"We're now applying for authorization by the Ministry of Public Health so that we can expand our production to meet national or even international demand, so that more drug addicts can benefit from this Chinese prescription."

According to the latest statistics, there are 500 drug-addiction treatment centers across China. As the oldest and largest, the Kunming center enjoys a reputation for its effective treatments. It now combines rehabilitation, education, scientific research and *626* production as well as the medical treatment of drug addiction. Since its establishment, it has successfully helped more than 12,000 addicts back to normal life.

The center is often on the itinerary of government officials, drug-fighting experts and scholars visiting the province. Many delegates, from more than 80 countries, spoke highly of the work they saw, some of them dubbing the facility "the world's No.1 drug treatment center."

The *626* capsule has obviously been central to the center's noteworthy success and gaining of worldwide regard. Quite a few overseas visitors have proposed cooperation with the center on the further development of this capsule and other potential cures.

In March 1996, four senior officials from the center and the city's Public Security Bureau were invited to tour the United States. There, the Chinese delegation signed a letter of intent with the Drug Study Center of Miami University. The US side agreed to fund a series of studies to be made at the Kunming center and to arrange for clinical trials of the 626 at the "Safe Port" Drug Addiction Treatment Center in Key West, Florida.

Regarding future stages of the capsule's development, Pan says researchers will focus their attention in two areas: further purification, thus enabling lower effective dosages to be made, and to make the prescription a cure for psychological as well as physical addiction.

Relapse Problem

This dual approach, he says, stems from recognition that the relapse rate of addicts who have kicked their habit is still very high. A 1995 post-cure survey reveals that the relapse rate of addicts treated at the Kunming center was as high as 75 percent.

Pan says: "Relapses are obviously no good to patients, and they are minuses for our efforts."

There are various reasons for relapse, many of them beyond the control of treatment centers, which calls for efforts from society.

For instance, patients lead a full life inside the center and cannot find drugs there, recalls Miss Cao, a former taxi driver.

"You don't miss the drugs at the center," she says. "But once you are out and have nothing to do, you naturally meet up with the drug addicts you once knew — then you are in danger of becoming hooked again."

While it is hard for the treatment center to check such negative associations, Pan says, "we must try to leave withdrawn patients with some kind of a drug-resistance effect so that they feel sick whenever they think of using drugs — only then will there be a chance of effecting a large number of permanent cures."

When that dream is realized, drug abuse will be eradicated. But in the meantime 626 gives addicts a chance to kick their habits. The rest is up to society. They must be accepted as recovered patients and be provided with social and family support to rebuild their shattered lives.

CHAPTER 14

A HAIR RAISER FOR WIG WEARERS

It's called 101 and percentage wise it's nearly that effective. After years of dedicated research, Zhao Zhangguang broke through on his 101st experiment to develop a preparation to reverse alopecia: baldness. Since then he has opened several pharmaceutical plants to produce his hair raiser for millions of prematurely bald people worldwide — much to the chagrin of wig manufacturers.

At 24, Wang Aiping began to suffer from a problem that would give most young women in China nightmares: hair loss. Within months she was completely bald. And the complaint was made all the more distressing in a country where females from their teens to their thirties pride themselves in sporting long, black shining hair.

But the problem was more than just cosmetic. Soon the baldness effected her work, her relationship. The distraught woman spent much of her time touring Beijing's hospitals in the hope of finding a cure. "I'd rather have died at the time," she recalled.

One hope after another faded. No medicine seemed to be able to regenerate hair growth. But Aiping kept looking and hoping.

The next hope, maybe like the many other useless ones, cropped up in April 1987 when Wang Aiping was browsing through the papers. A report stated that a Zhejiang doctor had opened a clinic in Beijing to specialize in the treatment of baldness. Moreover, it said many patients had been cured by the doctor's self-prepared herbal tincture.

With a mixture of hope and doubt, she set out to find the doctor. His name was Zhao Zhangguang, and he offered Wang Aiping two small bottles of a brown liquid and applied some of it to her bald head.

"On the second day I felt my head itching," Wang Aiping recalled, thinking that the medication might have triggered an allergic reaction. Another day passed and Aiping washed off a lot of scurf and yellowish deposit from her scalp. She was worried and went to see the doctor again. But she was surprised to see that Doctor Zhao was very pleased with the results, saying, "That's a good sign."

A few days later, Wang Aiping's bald scalp began to scab and sprout fine hair. In the next two months, normal hair started to grow. Six months later she had a thick head of hair and threw her wigs away — and then she got married. Today, with thick flowing hair, she is the mother of a six-year-old daughter and working as an accountant in a prestigious computer company in Beijing.

Wang Aiping is one among nearly six million patients, including 1.6 million foreigners, who have used the tincture.

The preparation is known as *101* Hair Regeneration Liniment. It can benefit those afflicted with both *pan-alopecia* (complete baldness) and *alopecia areata* (local baldness), male or female, regardless of age or race. The liniment has even managed to cure people who have been bald for 20 or more years.

According to available data, *101* has an effectiveness rate of 95 percent and a cure rate of 85 percent.

Zhao Zhangguang, 54, is chairman of the Beijing Zhangguang 101 Group. He says: "Millions of people worldwide are afflicted with baldness. I hope to market my *101* everywhere, helping bald people get rid of their wigs for good."

101st Experiment Breakthrough

Born in 1943 into a peasant family in Leqing County, in southeast China's Zhejiang Province, Zhao received only six years' education. An only son, he had to drop out of school to work in the family's fields.

In 1968, he visited a Hangzhou hospital — as a patient suffering from a skin disease. This experience later inspired him to become a "barefoot" doctor. He opened a clinic in his village, offering treatment for simple skin complaints. But he could not treat baldness.

An old medical saying stresses that baldness is one of the most difficult problems to treat. But Zhao refused to accept it.

He started his baldness study from scratch, knowing he was not the first to try in this field.

Zhao consulted experienced doctors of traditional Chinese medicine and herbalists. He read medical literature and studied the properties and effects of each herb.

He then made formulas and conducted experiments over and over again. He bought herbs with 5,000 yuan (equivalent to about US$1,200 then) in borrowed money. He even sold his house and pigs to fund his experiments. Soon his shabby-looking "laboratory" also served as his dwelling, crowded with pots and pans.

In his search for a herb that could quickly stimulate follicles to restore their hair-producing power without side effects, he applied herb sap to his skin. They often stung. To observe the response of patients in different age groups, he used his own father and son as guinea pigs. And he used his preparations on many bald-headed friends.

During a four-year experimental period he was constantly changing the preparation. He failed, strangely, exactly 100 times. But, at the 101st experiment, he was rewarded with a breakthrough. One of his best friends, Lin Guangnai, who suffered from baldness, returned one day exclaiming with excitement: "Zhangguang! My hair's growing!"

He named his herbal tincture *101*.

Later, Zhao offered free trial treatments to his bald-headed fellow villagers. Gradually, his *101* became known far and wide.

In the summer of 1983, the Zhejiang Workers Daily (newspaper) ran a story on Zhao; in 1984, he was invited to be honorary president of the Xiangyang Baldness Hospital in Zhengzhou, capital of Henan Province in central China, where Zhao later built a pharmaceutical plant with an annual production capacity of 200,000 bottles of *101* Hair Regeneration Liniment. In 1986 his preparation won a provincial prize in Henan.

This success caught the attention of leaders at the Ministry of Civil Affairs in Beijing. Representatives were sent to invite Zhao to Beijing, where the ministry wanted to fund a one-million yuan project to build a plant to produce *101*.

The manufacture of *101* takes two to three weeks. Initially, 20 rare medicinal herbs are combined. Then the mixture is blended with alcohol for about two weeks. The final process is dilution to remove alcoholic odor.

The liniment can keep the skin in a state of hyperaemia and improve blood circulation, which is essential for hair growth.

More Inventions

"But *101* cannot cure all forms of baldness, such as senile *alopecia seborrheica* in an advanced stage, or pseudo-baldness," says Zhao, who is not satisfied with his treatment of these conditions.

Zhao later developed *101-A*, which was put on test in five hospitals in Beijing in 1989. Designed especially to treat *alopecia* (a disease characterized by hair fallout with excessive secretion of skin fat), the new product is made from a new formula, quite different from that of *101*. It received formal approval for public use from the Ministry of Public Health in 1992.

Other 101 products Zhao has developed include *101-D* for different types of hair fallout, especially *alopecia seborrheica*; *101-E* for acne (comedo), *101 Fubao* for inflammatory acne and dermatitis; *101-F* for *alopecia seborrheica*, especially in its middle and late stages; *101 Xunxunbai*, a medical powder to cure freckles, nourish skin and smooth wrinkles; and *101* Shampoo that generally makes hair healthy and stops it from falling out.

An new auxiliary product, *102*, is now available, also to help prevent hair from falling out. It can be used with *101* or *101-A* for improved results.

For his inventions, Dr. Zhao Zhangguang has won seven gold medals including ones at invention fairs in Brussels, Geneva, Paris and New York.

More Production, Wider Service

The Zhangguang Group currently has four pharmaceutical factories turning out about two million bottles of *101* products a year.

The Beijing factory was the first to produce *101*-series tincture, having been in operation since April, 1987. It has advanced extracting equipment and a highly efficient bottling line.

Meanwhile, Zhao's group has set up consulting service departments, or "dermatology clinics," in different parts of the country.

The first such clinic opened for treatment in April 1987 in Beijing. With 20 doctors and staff members, the clinic receives about 160 patients a day, out of more than 300 who go there to seek advice as well as buy *101* products.

News about the remarkable effect of the *101*-series medicine has attracted many foreigners with baldness or balding problems.

To meet this demand, an International Rehabilitation Tourism Center has been set up in Beijing's Jinsong Hospital offering treatment to foreigners suffering from baldness. It is a joint venture: Zhao Zhangguang provides knowhow and medicine, Jinsong Hospital the facilities and medical personnel, while CITIC (China International Trust and Investment Corporation) Travel Co. makes travel arrangements.

But there is no need to travel all the way to China for *101* treatment. The group's products are exported to more than 40 countries and regions. To make distribution more reliable, the Zhao Zhangguang U.S. Corporation was established, as were branch offices in Japan and many European Union countries.

An official trade channel was established between Japan and the Zhangguang Group in April 1996 when the Osaka Municipal Government granted formal approval for importing the *101* tincture.

"On the whole, exports have continued to rise," says Zhao Zhangguang. "This has resulted from satisfactory services and publicity efforts as well as from the high reputation and good quality of the products."

Counterfeiting Problem

High demand for *101* has prompted profiteers to stockpile the product in an attempt to artificially create shortages and drive market prices up. For example, one bottle of *101* could be sold for US$100 on the black market in the mid-1980s, at a time when its recommended retail price was only US$20.

As demand for *101* keeps increasing, counterfeit *101* has reared its ugly head. Many buyers are tricked into thinking they have bought the real thing. But they soon find out it's fake. Zhao is very concerned about such malpractices, since they not only distress the sufferer and customer, but also damage the reputation of *101*.

Zhao has brought hope and hair to millions of bald people worldwide. But he won't rest on such laurels. "There are so many more bald people out there," he says. To spread his treatment, he plans to open clinics in all of China's provinces and regions, and all major cities of the world.

FOR RELEVANT ILLUSTRATIONS, SEE Figs. 24-27.

CHAPTER 15

SOUTH CHINA'S PHARMACEUTICAL INSTITUTION

The Hu Qing Yu Tang medicine store in Hangzhou, Zhejiang Province, epitomizes all that is good about Chinese medicine: expert practitioners, quality, traditional materials and a reliable service backed by more than a century's experience. Since 1874, citizens of Hangzhou have placed their utmost faith in the store, whose fame and reputation stretches much further afield, making Hu Qing Yu Tang a national institution.

When it came into being in the city of Hangzhou, Zhejiang Province, more than 120 years ago, it was no different from thousands of other Chinese herbal medicine stores scattered across the width and breadth of the land. But within a few years, it had thrived into a business giant that others could only admire.

Nowadays as a saying goes, the best drug store in the country's north is *Tong Ren Tang* in Beijing's Qianmen area, and that in the south *Hu Qing Yu Tang*, or "Mr. Hu's Prosperous Store."

Founded in 1874 by a wealthy merchant called Hu Xueyan, *Hu Qing Yu Tang* is a traditional store that originally sold drugs produced in a backyard workshop. In the 1950s, the store was turned into a state-owned complex. Much has happened in its 123-year-long history, including political turbulences and ups and downs in business turnovers. But the store has kept expanding its business and its age-old popularity has remained unchallenged. It is a success story that has inspired the sick to travel from afar for prescriptions.

Historians and those in traditional Chinese medical circles attribute the store's success to its founder's shrewd management and its traditionally near-fastidious demand for product quality.

Customer Care

Hu's shrewdness can be best illustrated by some stories that have been handed down from generation to generation both inside and outside *Hu Qing Yu Tang*. One tale recalls about how Hu selected the first manager for his store-workshop.

There were three candidates. The first one promised to earn 100,000 taels of silver in the first year after opening to business. The second one suggested aiming for small profits in the first two years — big money could be made from the third year onwards. The third candidate, however, said that in order to build fame for *Hu Qing Yu Tang*, it should first run at a loss for three consecutive years before seeking big profits. Hu chose the third candidate on the spot.

So in the first three years, the new manager Yu Xiuchu practiced the art of losing money. He invested money on building up the store's image and promoting its business. One thing he did was to send out the store's staff to the street to distribute drugs free of charge at weekends and during festival times. In summer, he would ask his staff to prepare herbal tea for customers, local residents and pedestrians to refresh them, again free of charge.

These charitable acts made a good impression on local people, but to win them over as frequent customers Mr. Hu knew he had to offer an excellent service and top quality products.

Unlike Western drugs, a traditional Chinese prescription is often composed of more than a dozen ingredients derived from herbs and animals. Some of these ingredients are rare and expensive, but when mixed together, only the most experienced in the processing of Chinese medicinal herbs can tell one ingredient from another. So the purchaser must trust the drug dealer and hope he does not cheat him.

Since it is natural that people would question a new drug dealer's honesty in its service, *Hu Qing Yu Tang* adopted "no cheating" as its business principle. The two characters *Jie Qi* written by Hu Xueyan were even inscribed on a board and were hung on the wall of the manager's office. The board is still hanging there today.

Another principle the store has adhered to is high quality. In preparing herbal medicines, achieving high quality is easier said than done. "It is actually extremely complicated," asserted Tang Changhua, a senior manager who has spent 20 years at *Hu Qing Yu Tang* Pharmaceutical Factory, as the store is named today.

The raw herbs should first be hand-picked to eliminate all foreign substances, then washed, sliced or ground. Then they should go through various processes including soaking, boiling, steaming, baking, extracting, filtering, mixing, stoving and shaping. Very often, each ingredient of a prescription is prepared separately by a different method before the mixing and finishing processes.

Hu Qing Yu Tang produces more than 300 medicines and tonic products in 13 forms, such as pills, powders, tinctures, oral liquids, instant drinks and capsules. Producing this range of medicines involves the collection and use of more than 2,000 kinds of herbs, minerals and medicinal materials from animals.

To ensure product quality, the old workshop used a gold slice and a silver pot for the making of *Zixuedan*, an external-use pill for treating miliary vesicle. Ingredients boiled in the pot were said to retain greater medicinal properties.

Sometimes an ancient prescription sets such strict demands on raw materials that it seems more magically-based in its function than scientifically-based. Hence *Hu Qing Yu Tang* has stuck to original instructions concerning the preparation of prescriptions for the sake of quality.

Time-Honored Methods

Tradition is carefully adhered to, as demonstrated in the making of the *Biwendan* pill, which has proved effective in preventing pestilence and malaria.

One of the 74 ingredients in the pill is a special kind of lizard, which has a bright yellow line on its back and is found only in the hills near Lingyin Temple in Hangzhou. Although lizards found elsewhere appear similar, even under chemical and spectral analysis, the prescription allows no replacement.

"We once made replacements, but strangely pills made from other lizards were really less effective," said Deng Liyi, head of the pharmaceutical institute run by *Hu Qing Yu Tang*.

Most prescriptions at *Hu Qing Yu Tang* come from the secret royal pharmacopoeia of the Southern Song Dynasty (1127-1270) and some can even be traced back to Han Dynasty (206BC-220AD). The rest are collected from folk remedies, a distinct variation from Beijing's *Tong Ren Tang* whose official prescriptions largely served the imperial court.

"People have a strong faith in us, because we've done our best to remain traditional in terms of prescribing and dispensing Chinese medicine," Tang Changhua claimed.

Human Resources

To preserve traditional merits such as processing techniques, old masters at *Hu Qing Yu Tang* today have not only compiled a guide which must be read by young dispensing chemists, but they have also continued the old practice of employing apprentices, believing it to be a good way of passing on their skills. A college graduate can be promoted to the position of senior dispensing pharmacist after serving a three-year apprenticeship.

Such promotion may sound easily achievable, but in reality the reward is well-deserved. Processing skills, crucial to product quality, are difficult to command and some of them are kept secret.

"Japan used to claim that within 15 years it was going to better China in the making of herbal medicines, and it did succeed in some ways," said Tang Changhua. "It has developed impressive manufacturing and testing machines, but it cannot acquire our traditional and exclusive processing skills," he said. Hence the position of traditional Chinese medicine remains unchallenged.

Machines for example are quick, but they cannot replace a traditionally-trained dispensing pharmacist. Take slicing for example, which is the most common and basic task in any traditional medicine store in China.

The thinner a herb is sliced, the better it releases its medicinal effects during the boiling process. A typical method of testing a worker's slicing skill at *Hu Qing Yu Tang* is to give him a betel nut, derived from a palm tree of the same name, and see how many slices he can make: the standard for a "pass" is 108. But a machine can only produce about a dozen slices out of a betel nut. Hence machines are not used for slicing.

Another testing job — which is very often beyond the capability of machines and instruments — is evaluating wild ginseng, an expensive tonic medicine. Tang likens the evaluation process in terms of skill required to that of tea- or wine-tasting. "Instruments can tell you something, but not everything, and often not the most important things," he said.

However, modern technology is applied where possible. The testing of product quality, for instance, used to rely on workers' experience, who could tell by the sight and smell of the product. Now with the introduction of testing instruments, workers are freed from the exhausting job.

Production lines that produce herbal medicines in the forms of oral liquids, tablets and capsules have been imported from the West. Last year, a preparation workshop was built with equipment supplied by a British plant and Sino-foreign joint ventures. Machines now perform about 60 percent of the total labor at *Hu Qing Yu Tang*.

With traditional skills and modern technology joining hands, *Hu Qing Yu Tang* has kept expanding its business, which in 1996 reached 77 million yuan (US$9.3 million) in sales, up from just 10 million yuan (US$1.2 million) in the early 1980s.

Tang attributes the growth to their efforts in opening new markets outside China in recent years. He said that *Hu Qing Yu Tang* was the first pharmaceutical factory in the country to export a Chinese herbal drug. But in the past, he added, their exports were limited to Southeast Asia and they could not enter Western markets, due to Westerners' ignorance of the tenets and effects of traditional Chinese medicine.

Business improved in the early 90s when *Hu Qing Yu Tang* began to expand its exports to Japan, South Korea, the United States and Europe. It even opened a joint-venture enterprise in Ukraine to produce herbal medicines, using Chinese technologies and local medicinal materials.

At present *Hu Qing Yu Tang* is targeting more markets. Tang said more and more Westerners are discovering the wonders of Chinese medicine for themselves, "which parallels the world trend of returning to natural foods, drinks, lifestyles and finally, medicines."

In fact, even on its native soil, traditional Chinese medicine is booming. All over the country, free medical care once provided by the state via employers is being replaced by social medical insurance as China restructures its economy. And because people have to foot their own medical bills they tend to prefer herbal drugs which, though often slower to function, are less expensive and less likely to induce side effects.

To grasp this opportunity, *Hu Qing Yu Tang* has shifted its production focus from tonics to medicine. In the past, its tonics sold better on the domestic market and sales thereof accounted for 70 percent of the total. Now it is vice versa with medicine taking up 83 percent of total sales.

"In the future," said Liu Jun, general manager of *Hu Qing Yu Tang*, "the century-old pharmaceutical business is going to pay more attention to the development of new products, because old prescriptions are being produced by too many pharmaceutical factories and therefore it is very difficult to organize large-scale commercial production."

Two or three new products are developed at *Hu Qing Yu Tang* every year. *Xifeining*, a medicine developed to relieve the symptoms of silicosis and first marketed five years ago, has found a market-niche and is a big cash earner.

To further expand its production capability, *Hu Qing Yu Tang* is constructing new production buildings at a new location in Hangzhou. They will be completed in 1998.

General Manager Liu is quite ambitious, and he has reasons to be. "More than a century has passed, and yet *Hu Qing Yu Tang* is still flourishing in its image of being the medicine king in China's south. We are proud of our traditional legacy and we are determined to make Mr. Hu's Prosperous Store even more prosperous."

FOR RELEVANT ILLUSTRATIONS, SEE Figs. 28-30.

CHAPTER 16

A HERBAL SWIPE AT MALARIA

Ancient Chinese first aid notes written 16 centuries ago, Handbook of Prescriptions for Emergencies, recommended the use of a bitter, cool-tasting plant to relieve malarial symptoms and heat exhaustion. Pressurized by the growing ineffectiveness of quinine as an anti-malarial drug, researchers in Shanghai, working from their historical lead, have developed artemether, regarded by the World Health Organization as the most effective medicine to combat the mosquito-born parasite.

On the threshold of a new century malaria, which has long plagued man living or traveling in the tropics and sub-tropics, continues to kill two million throughout the world each year. Half of all annual malaria victims are children in Africa.

Since the 1960s, malaria has been increasingly difficult to control since the malaria-causing sporazoan parasite, genus plasmodium, has grown to resist century-old quinine and related drugs.

But there is a new hope: artemether, a derivative of *Qing Hao Su* (*Artemisinin*), an antimalarial substance extracted from the medicinal herb *Qing Hao* (*Artemisia Annua Linn*). It has been jointly developed by the Shanghai Institute of Materia Medica under the Chinese Academy of Sciences and the Kunming Pharmaceutical Corporation

(KPC).

The World Health Organization (WHO) has confirmed that artemether is the best remedy for malaria, a parasitic disease mostly seen in tropical and subtropical climes.

"Artemether remarkably brings about cures for various types of malarias, such as malignant malaria, marked by recurrence of spasms in less than 48 hours; vivax malaria, marked by recurrences of spasms at 48-hour intervals, and quinoline-derived-antimalarial-drug-resistant malignant malaria," says the KPC president Li Nangao. "It is also a very effective schizonticide (killer) of malarial parasites in the erythrocyte, or vertebrate blood-cell stage."

The KPC now exports the new drug, in the form of injection and capsules, and artemether raw materials to 27 malarial-prevalent countries and regions. In 1995, the corporation earned US$1.2 million from export trade. While declining to disclose annual output, Li says that KPC is manufacturing artemether drugs in quantities large enough to support treatment for all the 200 million victims of malaria in the world.

Compound benflumetol, which is a combination of artemether and benflumetol, is another new achievement of collaboration between the KPC, the Chinese People's Liberation Army Medical Science Academy, the CITIC Technology Company, and Ciba-Geigy Ltd. of Switzerland. Benflumetol is a medication developed by the PLA academy to treat malaria, but its function used to be limited since it takes effect rather slowly. Therefore it was of little use in cases of acute nature.

"Since artemether is especially effective during the first few days of its administration, and benflumetol is extraordinarily efficacious some time after being taken, a mixture of the two — compound benflumetol — is a more-certain cure for malaria and is less likely to be proceeded by relapses within 28 days of commencing treatment," Li says confidently.

The new drug is now being reviewed by the Ministry of Public Health, he says.

Tasting bitter and cool, *Artemisia Annua Linn*, the wild plant, was used as a medication for summer heat discomfort and malaria in China as early as 1,600 years ago. *Handbook of Prescriptions for Emergencies* by Ge Hong (281-341) and *Compendium Materia Medica* by Li Shizhen (1518-1593) record its properties. Today, some village folk are still using the plant for treating malaria.

In the early 1970s, the Chinese Ministry of Public Health set up a think tank and research group at the Shanghai Institute of Materia Medica to search for an alternative to quinine for the prevention of malaria.

For historical reasons the researchers started with *Artemisia Annua Linn*. "At first we got Artemisinin," recalls Zhang Chucheng, biochemist research chief of the program. "But through tests we found that it still left a recurrence rate of about 50 percent — it just shocked, rather than killed, the plasmodium parasites. We went further on with our research and synthesized more than 100 derivatives from Artemisinin. And we tested them one by one on animals. In March 1976 we derived artemether, a lipid solution, which we called *Hao Jia Mi* in Chinese. We found it an ideal solution."

Clinical trials proved that artemether, with a low toxicant, is the most effective anti-malarial compound developed so far, says Zhu Dayuan, a research fellow with the research group of the Shanghai Institute of Materia Medica. "By March 1980 the Ministry of Public Health initially designated it as the top choice to combat malaria."

Then the institute cooperated with the KPC (previously known as the Kunming Pharmaceutical Factory) in pre-production trials of artemether injection, finally transferring the technical know-how to the factory. The KPC is now the sole manufacturer of artemether in China.

"Compared with quinine, artemether acts more quickly to reduce feverish symptoms and eliminate parasites," says Prof. Wang Tongyin of the Epidemic Prevention Medical Science Department of the Kunming Medical College based in the capital of Yunnan, who began to put artemether into clinical use in 1979. "And it induces no adverse reactions such as nausea, dizziness or miscarriage as quinine does frequently, although it may also have some slight side effects such as transient fever or transient decrease in reticulocyte count."

Dr. Che Ligang, former director of the Yunnan Provincial Malaria Prevention and Cure Center based in Simao, southern Yunnan, an area which used to be so severely plagued with malaria that it was nicknamed "City of Death," claims that the clinical cure rate of artemether has been 100 percent since he started using it at his center in 1984.

"The recurrence rate is a little more than five percent, and that only happens in cases of malignant malaria," says the doctor who joined the artemether experiment program in 1978 and has been working with malaria victims in Simao for 35 years.

Clinical trials of the herbal injection on 1,088 malarial cases in five of China's provinces in the late 1970s also showed a 100 percent effective rate. Follow-up visits to 343 malignant malaria patients revealed a radical cure rate of more than 90 percent.

Safety

Moreover, artemether proves to be safe in curing pregnant women inflicted with malignant malaria.

A Burmese woman, Kayenki, was five-months pregnant when she contracted malignant malaria and was sent to the nearby Zhangfeng Township Hospital in Yunnan for emergency treatment. Prof. Wang Tongyin treated her with artemether. Three days later Kayenki was well enough to be released from hospital. A few months later she gave birth to a healthy baby.

"Malignant malaria is fatal for pregnant women," Wang says. "And the known treatments using quinine often cause miscarriages or still births. That's why we say artemether is miraculous."

Between 1976 and 1980, Wang conducted a survey on six women who were 17-27 weeks' pregnant and suffering from malaria. They all lived in Luxi and Longchuan counties, Dehong Prefecture, Yunnan. Wang cured all of them with artemether injections, and made a long-term follow-up study on the labors and subsequent fertility of the mothers, and growth and congenital deformity, if any, of their children.

"No adverse reaction was found on the fetuses. No deformity was caused to the babies. No negative influence was observed on the development and mentality of the children, or on the subsequent fertility of the mothers," Wang stated.

After two decades' efforts by Chinese scientists to search for a quinine substitute, artemether finally became known to the world in 1981, when an international conference on artemisinin and its derivatives was held in Beijing under the auspices of the United Nations Development Program, World Bank and WHO. Dr. N. Anand, director of the Central Drug Research Institute of India who chaired the conference, praised Chinese scientists for their "significant discovery" of the new compound with what he called a unique chemical structure, which has no similarity to any known anti-malarials.

After further pharmacological and toxicological experiments and clinical trials, the Ministry of Public Health officially defined the artemether injection and two other artemisinin injections as "new antimalarials specifically for treatment of various critical malarias and for emergency treatment of cerebral malaria" in September 1987.

WHO Recognition

In 1990, the WHO recognized artemether as the most effective antimalaria drug in the world, and allocated US$2 million for its clinical trials in several malaria- rampant countries, including Nigeria, Kenya and Malawi in Africa, Thailand and Vietnam in Asia, and Brazil in South America.

Trial feedback was positive and encouraging. According to Prof. Sornchai Looareesuwan of Mahidol's Faculty of Tropical Medicine in Thailand, artemether's cure rate there is more than 94 percent. In Brazil, the government approved the importation of 500,000 catheters of artemether injection from China in December 1990, having tried the first 60,000 tubes of the injection, a gift to the Brazilian people from visiting Chinese President Yang Shangkun earlier that year.

The KPC then invested 32 million yuan (US$3.9 million) in building a new workshop for manufacturing artemether drugs and importing advanced production line and test equipment from Germany, the United States and Japan.

After close inspection of the workshop in 1990 and 1991, a group of WHO experts, including Dr. D. Davidson and Dr. H. Pang, acknowledged that the workshop had attained a standard of quality assurance consistent with Good Manufacturing Practices (GMP).

To promote international sales of its artemether medications, the KPC has entered into cooperation with Rhone Poulenc Rorer Company (RPR) of France, one of the country's top ten medical companies, and a leading manufacturer and seller of anti-malarial drugs in the world. RPR is now acting as the general agent for the KPC's artemether products throughout the world.

The artemether inventors and manufacturer have created several firsts for China's pharmaceutical industry. The drug is the country's first to be listed by WHO in the International Pharmacopoeia and Essential Drugs. Also, it is the first in China to have its trademark registered abroad. Out of the 40 countries where registration has been completed, 27 are importing or selling artemether drugs produced by the KPC. Meanwhile, the Kunming corporation has applied for a patent, also a first among Chinese pharmaceutical producers, to protect its invention of artemether in 68 countries and regions. Twenty-two have so far granted patents.

Other Applications

While artemether was developed to deal with malaria, Zhang Chucheng and his colleagues have discovered that it is actually capable of killing many kinds of viruses, and can even alleviate AIDS symptoms.

"When used for AIDS cases, artemether proved effective in controlling the infection of an HIV-related bacteria called *can didaal bicans*, which is a terminal symptom of AIDS, and in prolonging the patient's survival," says Dr. Wu Yunchao of the Yunnan Provincial People's Hospital. During his service as a member of the Fourth Chinese Medical Team providing aid to Uganda from 1989-1991, Wu applied the anti-malarial drug to 144 AIDS patients suffering from thrush.

"It was the first time artemether was applied to AIDS cases with the *can didaal bicans* infection," Dr. Wu says. "Its effect on those cases was evident, but further study is needed before we can say it is very effective for the deadly disease."

To date *Artemisia Annua Linn* is found to grow only in China, particularly in Yunnan, Sichuan, Guizhou and Guangxi.

Strangely enough, he says, when grown abroad from seeds collected in China, the plant becomes much less effective as an anti-malarial cure, "for the natural environment under which it grows is much, much different."

Zhang is therefore confident that China will remain the sole manufacturer of artemether, even in the next century.

His confidence in artemether is enhanced by results from his research work in the United States. "Plasmodium parasite will be unable to develop a strong resistance to artemether in the next five decades," he says.

FOR RELEVANT ILLUSTRATIONS, SEE Figs. 31 & 32.

CHAPTER 17

SCALP ACUPUNCTURE: THERAPY CLOSE TO THE SITE OF STROKES

The seemingly logical application of acupuncture on the heads of stroke-induced victims was only made in the most-recent chapter of the treatment's long history. Chen Daoyi has identified needling lines and designed an electrical stimulator to turn inserted needles at speed, thus achieving a greater therapeutic effect than that induced by hand rotation.

In China, severe disabilities resulting from strokes are commonly treated by traditional Chinese medicine, *qigong* and massage, but acupuncture applied to the scalp has also brought relief and even cure to sufferers.

As the description suggests, scalp acupuncture is implemented by applying needles to the top part of the head. However, their precise place of application, their angle of insertion, depth of penetration and rotation rate, makes the treatment a particularly exacting one to administer.

The method dates back to the early 1960s, when it was used in Shanxi Province, but it was perfected for clinical use by Doctor Chen Daoyi, 61, now director of the Scalp Acupuncture Hospital in Wangjiang County, Anhui Province. Since 1981 he has treated 1,640 stroke victims, and others afflicted by brain diseases, with scalp acupuncture. Ninety-three percent of the patients showed markedly alleviated states of disability and 61.5 percent were diagnosed as being cured of their paralysis and speech defects.

"The therapy essentially correlates traditional Chinese acupuncture with modern theories of neuroanatomy, since both postulate that connections exist between specific areas of the scalp and brain, and elsewhere in the body," explains Jiang Dashu, director of the neurology department of the Acupuncture Institute under the Academy of Traditional Chinese Medicine.

"Therefore it is therapeutically effective to needle specific areas on the head in order to treat problems in those parts of the body governed by them," Jiang says.

Based on this theory, Chen has identified "needling lines" — imaginary lines which connect two acupoints — on the top part of the head, which he targets by the insertion of his needles.

On the forehead are seven such lines, existing as three pairs and one single line. On the top of the head are four pairs and one single line; on each temple is a pair of lines, while on the occiput, or back of the head, are two pairs and one single line.

"Altogether six single and ten pairs of acupoints are involved," Chen says.

"Each line corresponds to a certain part of the body," he says, "for instance, two pairs of the lines on the temples are important for the treatment of the paralysis of upper and lower limbs, as well as loss of speech."

Chen uses capillary needles of 0.32-0.38mm in diameter and 50-66mm in length. "I insert the needle precisely at an angle of 30 degrees to the scalp, and to a depth of 33-50mm," he says. Then an electric stimulator is used to rotate the needle at a rate of 130 to 400 revolutions per minute, according to the demands of the particular condition.

Chen designed the stimulator himself and started to use it on patients in 1986. "Before that I had to rotate the needle by hand — it was extremely exhausting," he says. "I had to stand as still as possible throughout a session, just twirling the needles with my fingers until the desired number of revolutions had been achieved — it usually took about 30 minutes."

With the stimulator, the doctor has not only freed himself and other practitioners from that painstaking labor. Use of the stimulator allows the practitioner to control the rate of needle revolution, thereby introducing a further variable which can be altered according to the

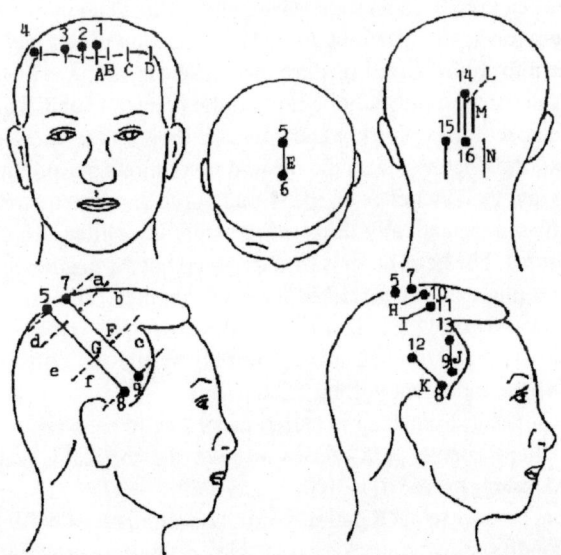

Acupoints and needling lines commonly used in scalp acupuncture therapy.

Acupoints
1 *Shenting* (single)
2 *Meichong*
3 *Toulinqi*
4 *Touwei*
5 *Baihui* (single)
6 *Qianding* (single)
7 *Qianshencong* (single)
8 *Qubin*
9 *Xuanli*
10 *Tongtian*
11 *Zhengying*
12 *Shuaigu*
13 *Hanyan*
14 *Qiangjian*
15 *Yuzhen*
16 *Naohu*

Needling Lines
A) Mid forehead line (single)
B) Side forehead line No. 1
C) Side forehead line No. 2
D) Side forehead line No. 3
E) Mid crown line (single)
F) Front crown-temple line
 a) movement of leg
 b) movement of arm
 c) movement of face, speech
G) Back crown-temple line
 d) sensation of leg
 e) sensation of arm
 f) sensation of face, speech
H) Side crown line No. 1
I) Side crown line No. 2
J) Front temple line
K) Back temple line
L) Mid occiput line (single)
M) Side occiput line
N) Side sub-occiput line

needs of each individual case. Meanwhile, Chen can concentrate on selecting the acupoints along the selected needling lines, helping the patient into the required posture, and inserting the needles one by one. A nurse then puts a hoop around the patient's head. This holds both the needles in position and connects them to the stimulator.

Next, the doctor selects the desired revolutions per minute (rpm) setting and then switches on the stimulator to start the treatment.

A timer automatically turns off the stimulator after two minutes' revolutions. The head hoop is then removed but the needles are left in place on the head for a further 10 to 20 minutes. The procedure is usually repeated twice before the needles are finally removed.

"The stronger the sensation reported by the patient, the more effective the treatment will be," Chen says.

The rotation frequency is varied according to each case, he says. For a patient recently paralyzed by a stroke, the rpm dial is set towards the maximum, from 310 to 400.

"That's because such patients still have strength to battle against their conditions," the doctor says. "Fast rotation may stimulate the scalp vigorously, promoting blood circulation and restoring the function of the affected limbs to normal."

For the most serious of cases, such as paralysis due to cerebral hemorrhages, needle rotation is set at a lower frequency, between 100 and 200 rpm.

"Lower frequencies aim to galvanize the cortical cells corresponding to the unaffected parts first, and so improve circulation of qi, vital energy, within the body, which may ultimately activate the paralyzed parts," Chen says.

For patients in less-serious condition, he says, a balanced pattern of rotation is used, with a medium setting of 200 to 300 rpm being selected.

Chen Daoyi explains that the electric stimulator reinforces the therapeutic effect of scalp acupuncture. It "induces a stronger needling response" than that effected by manual rotation. It maintains a much more precise needling angle and more accurate rotation frequency, thus producing more even stimulation. After the use of the stimulator, the cure rate among scalp acupuncture-treated patients improved by more than 20 percent.

It seems from Chen's statistics that his therapy is most effective when applied to cases of cerebral thrombosis and cerebral angiitis. He boasts a cure rate of 70 percent in these areas. With cases of cerebral hemorrhage, cerebral embolism, brain contusion and sequelae of meningitis, his treatment has achieved a cure rate of 51 percent.

Wu Antao, an engineer with the Design & Research Institute for Chemical Mines under the Ministry of Chemical Industry in Lianyungang, Jiangsu Province, had the left side of his body paralyzed after a stroke ten years ago. He was bedridden for more than one year before he turned to Chen's scalp acupuncture therapy.

After 12 months' treatment, Wu said he could raise his left arm and walk with ease. Now a senior engineer with his institute, the 55-year-old man had little to complain about, apart from a leg strain — which happened while running! "Chen's scalp acupuncture not only helped me get rehabilitated physically but also improved my thinking capability," said Wu.

Wu Antao recalled that when the doctor twirled the needles he felt "some soreness". Such a reaction, called *De Qi*, or roughly "arresting the vital energy," indicates that a therapeutic effect is being induced, according to Chen. Continuous rotating creates sensations of warmth, numbness, or spasmodic contractions in the patient's paralyzed limbs.

Jin Xingrui, 61, a retired local postwoman, suffered a stroke in May, 1990. Her left side was paralyzed due to hypertension and cerebral thrombosis. She was hospitalized for two weeks before deciding to move over to Chen's hospital.

Just three days later she could walk 20 meters without support. After her first course of treatment, which lasted 15 days, she was able to walk 40 meters by herself. By the end of the second course, Jin could walk more than 500 meters and lift her once-paralyzed left arm upright. Moreover, fingers once stiffened could function well to hold things, lace up shoes and button coats.

"Most patients come to me within a few weeks or months of being attacked, but I've treated some who were bedridden for one year," Chen says, stressing that the therapeutic effect of scalp acupuncture is at its greatest if administered as soon as possible after the stroke.

Most of his patients show improvement after two or three courses of treatment, and there is a 3- to 5-day interval between courses. Normally the function of the paralyzed limbs gets restored before that of speech, while the lower limbs lead the upper ones in recovery. The fingers take the longest time to restore to normal, Chen says.

The patient is required to do exercises to promote rehabilitation as soon as his paralyzed limbs become mobile. "You can't totally rely on the doctor to get fully recovered," he says.

Located in the seat of Wangjiang County which lies about 250km west of Nanjing, Chen's hospital has more than 100 beds. In recent years, patients have come for treatment from the United States, United Kingdom, Bangladesh, Hong Kong and Taiwan.

Scalp acupuncture was recognized as a valuable method for treating paralysis, loss of speech and other consequences of brain damage by the World Health Organization in 1984.

FOR RELEVANT ILLUSTRATION, SEE Fig. 33.

CHAPTER 18

ATTACKING THE PARASITIC CULPRIT OF ACNE

Acne disfigures, temporarily or permanently, some 130 million Chinese and countless other millions worldwide. Unlike most Western doctors, Zhao Zhongzhou believes the sole cause of the complaint to be a parasite called demodex. Eradicating its infestation of facial habitats, he stresses, is the essential step to give people blemish-free complexions.

Over the centuries, physicians have offered scores of theories to explain spotty faces, ranging from eating too much chocolate to citrus fruits, from apples to adolescence. But the stubborn red swellings remain on many faces.

Zhao Zhongzhou is believed to be one of the first doctors in the world who is capable of knocking spots off wherever they might be, after identifying the sole culprit: a parasite called *demodex*.

Zhao, 67, has 40 years' experience as a surgeon, initially in the People's Liberation Army, then in a hospital of an enterprise. He invented *Zhongzhou* Ointment and is now the chairman of the board of directors of Kunming *Zhongzhou* Pharmaceutical Corporation Limited based in Kunming, capital of southwest China's Yunnan Province.

With an invention patent granted by China's State Patent Office, the ointment wiped acne off the faces of 93.46 percent of 107 patients who took part in a clinical test in 1985-86.

Now, more than 100 acne rosacea clinics have opened in China. They exclusively use *Zhongzhou* Ointment for treating the ailment. A number of dermatologists working in the clinics say that many of their patients had suffered for 20 or 30 years from acarodermatitis, and had tried every medicinal ointment touted as being a cure, but to no avail. Their unpleasant symptoms subsided only after they took to *Zhongzhou* Ointment.

A survey of 2,723 acne cases, conducted at the Hospital Affiliated with the Military Medicine Academy in Beijing, No. 2 Hospital Affiliated with the Shenyang Medical College and six other clinics around the country, between March 1986 and October 1992, revealed an improvement rate of 99.7 percent and a cure rate of 93.39 percent. At a clinic in Zhangzhou, in southeast China's Fujian Province, the cure rate was as high as 96.22 percent.

Xiong Heping of the Xi'an Bakery and Confectionery in Shaanxi Province says that he used to have a red face covered with acne.

"I was very worried. I visited a number of hospitals in Xi'an and used dozens of bottles of a medicine said to be effective for acne rosacea. But I stayed spotty," Xiong says.

After using a few bottles of *Zhongzhou* Ointment in the fall of 1991, however, only two small red spots were left beside his nose. He felt sure that they would disappear if he continued to use the ointment. "*Zhongzhou* Ointment is miraculous," he proclaims.

The ointment consists of about eight Chinese and Western medicines such as sulphur, zinc oxide and Java brucea. It acts as a kind of germicide to kill *demodexes* on the skin of the face. "More often than not, most of the *demodexes* will be killed within a month," Zhao says.

Aside from killing *demodexes*, reducing inflammation and soothing itching which leads to pain — which is the main complaint about acarodermatitis apart from its unsightliness — the ointment also moistens the skin. After several weeks' use, patients can usually look in the mirror and see an unblemished facial appearance the likes of which they may have missed for years, or even decades.

And since the ointment is hormone-free and contains no poisonous substances such as lead, benzene or mercury, its long-term use will have no detrimental or side effects. And its ingredients are non-addictive.

Zhao says that acarodermatitis is a persistent ailment that many people suffer from throughout their lives. "The fact that few doctors acknowledge that *demodex* is the only cause of the ailment compounds difficulty in curing it," he says.

Over the past few years, Zhao says, researchers from many countries including the United States, New Zealand, Australia and China have been investigating the incidence of *demodicidosis* among the population. What they found was a conformity: each country reported an infection rate of approximately 60 percent, while the rate of incidence, mostly through contagion, was around 10 percent. As for rosacea alone, one of the two ailments caused by acarodermatitis, the occurrence rate was 2.44 percent.

"That means 130 million Chinese people are suffering from acarodermatitis — 30 million of them have red noses," Zhao says. "That's why I believe my work is so important."

The Parasite

Demodex is usually 100-200 microns long. In simple terms it's smaller than the tiniest insect but bigger than a germ. There are two types — the long and short. Parasitizing the facial sebaceous glands at an appropriate temperature, *demodexes* reproduce by a generation every 15 days. The adult *demodexes* die soon after the reproduction and the bodies rot and liquidate inside the sebaceous glands. Since *demodexes* spend all their lives inside the sebaceous glands, they physically and chemically affect the skin, reducing its immuno-competence, and causing allergic reactions in some parts of skin tissues, where red spots (acne) breaks out. This is sometimes known as adolescents' acne for obvious reasons.

"If not treated properly with correct medication, the inflammation will reoccur. In more serious cases, the epidermis, or the appearance of skin, will be permanently injured, scars resembling the texture of orange skin will be left, hair-follicle pores will be enlarged, and the skin will become thicker due to hyperplasia. Sometimes, the inflammation even leads to superfluous tumors or lumps, and red nose," Zhao explains.

What hinders the permeation of medicine is the membrane enclosing the eggs of *demodex*. "Therefore, patients are required to apply the ointment continuously, without any intervals, until a seborrhea test shows negative: that indicates a full recovery," Zhao says.

Generally, he says, victims of superficial *demodex* rosacea caused by long *demodex* should use the ointment for 60-80 days, while patients of deep *demodex* rosacea caused by short *demodex* should use the medicine for 90-120 days. The therapies must go on to the end "even if the symptom of inflammation disappears two to three weeks after first using the ointment."

Those who are found to have *demodex* existing in their skin but do not yet suffer from acarodermatitis may effectively prevent themselves contracting the disease by applying the ointment.

Zhao says he started thinking about finding ways to cure the skin disorder on the battleground of the War to Resist U.S. Aggression and Aid Korea (1950-53).

"I was a surgeon in the Chinese People's Volunteers in North Korea. A friend of mine, an officer, had a red nose. He earnestly appealed to me for help. I said I'd try," he recalls.

After numerous failures, Zhao developed an ointment which contained both traditional Chinese herbs and Western medicines, and, in a few months, he was delighted to find it cured his comrade of the rosacea.

"That was back in 1956," Zhao says. "I was fairly young, and curious. I asked myself 'Why not try the ointment on others and see if it also effects a cure?' "

So he did. From 1956-76, his cure rate remained about 80 percent, while the total rate of his ointment being effective to a reasonable degree approached 100 percent.

After demobilization in 1976, Zhao worked as a doctor and deputy director of Hospital No. 153 under the Ministry of Weaponry Industry. A worker in his 30s asked Zhao to rid him of rosacea. Zhao did it successfully. The worker was so pleased that he told the story to everyone he met. More and more sufferers sought the same treatment. Zhao worked to improve his ointment and enhance its cure rate.

By 1984, Zhao's treatment was in such high demand that he opened a special clinic in his hospital, where he treated the sufferers of acarodermatitis on Wednesdays and Fridays.

Before he retired in 1989, Zhao prepared his ointment in the dispensary of the hospital. His retirement, however, terminated that privilege. He had to think of finding a manufacturer.

In 1990, Zhao signed a contract with the Xinxiang People's

Pharmaceutical Factory based in Xinxiang, Henan Province. The ointment was named *Fu Man Ke Xing*, which means "killer of *demodexes*."

In September 1993, the ointment satisfied a panel of medical experts in Henan Provincial Public Health Bureau.

A year later, Zhao set up *Zhongzhou* Pharmaceutical Corporation Limited in Kunming. Having improved the production of the ointment, he renamed it *Zhongzhou* Ointment.

Zhao was a voluntary expert donating his ointment to those who needed it during Beijing's staging of the Asian Games in 1990.

In August 1991, the International Congress of New Drug Development in Seoul, South Korea, invited Zhao to present his thesis *Instruction of Zhao Zhongzhou's Ointment for Acne Rosacea*. The congress granted him an official product number of (91) P.D.-7 for his ointment.

In 1993, the ointment won a gold medal at the Fair of New Science and Technology Results and Patent Technology and Products, sponsored by the State Science and Technology Commission. In 1994, Zhao's ointment won another gold at the Fifth Asian and Pacific International Trade Fair.

Zhao feels it critical to stress that acarodermatitis is never a hereditary disease. "It is contagious," Zhao emphasizes. "Newborn babies have no *demodex*. They get it only after constant contact, for example by kissing, or sharing one towel, with those adults carrying *demodexes*."

He complains that prevention is neglected due to ignorance. "Doctors should tell people how to avoid being infected."

Zhao's target for 1997 is to turn out two million boxes of his ointment, and gain gross sales of 60 million yuan (US$7.2 million). It's a means to an end: to wipe out all acne.

FOR RELEVANT ILLUSTRATIONS, SEE Figs. 34-38.

CHAPTER 19

REMEDIES FROM FOREST AND FAMILY

Guizhou Province in southwest China boasts a huge assemblage of plants which are a vast source of medicinal materials for local nationalities in the region. Liao Hongyou is not unusual by the fact that he followed in his father's medicine-making footsteps, but he has made strides in popularizing what were once secret family cures to overcome an array of problems, especially in the area of bone fractures.

Xia Wei suffered from the painful after-effects of an accident he had in his infancy.

It could have happened to any mother, no matter how careful. With babe in arms, she stumbled while going downstairs. And before she could regain her balance her child had fallen and cut his head — badly. He was just 100 or so days old.

After the baby was rushed to a local hospital, the bleeding was stopped, and superficially at least Xia Wei's mother thought her son was in good health. Little did anyone know that the child had a fracture of the occipital bone (the back of his skull) and that it would remain that way, giving pain, for years to come.

The boy grew to be a weak child, his face wrinkled beyond his years, his body as frail as a baby's. His intellect was also lacking for

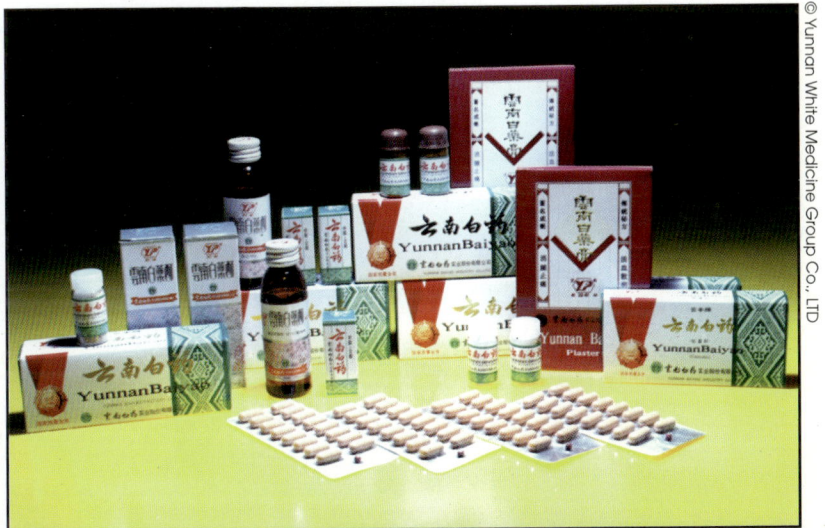

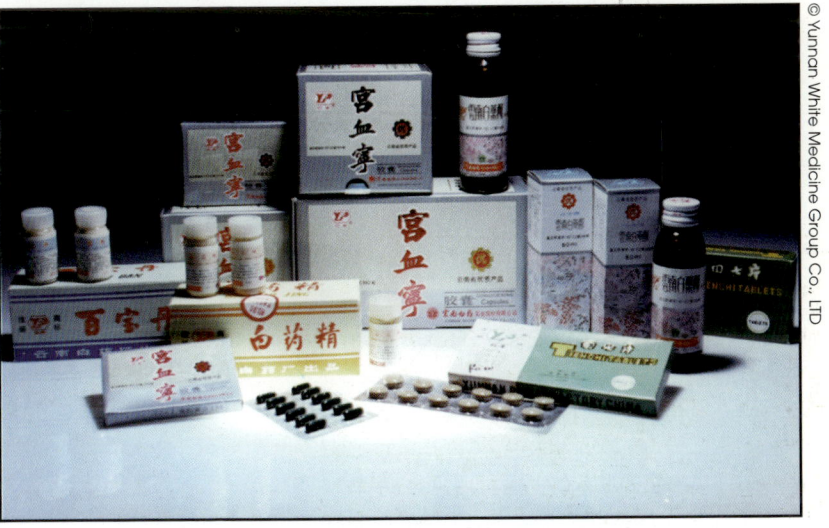

Fig.20 Different forms of White Medicine including powder and plasters, tablets and capsules, and tincture. *Gongxuening* capsules have proved effective in clinical tests for the treatment of intrauterine haemorrhaging.

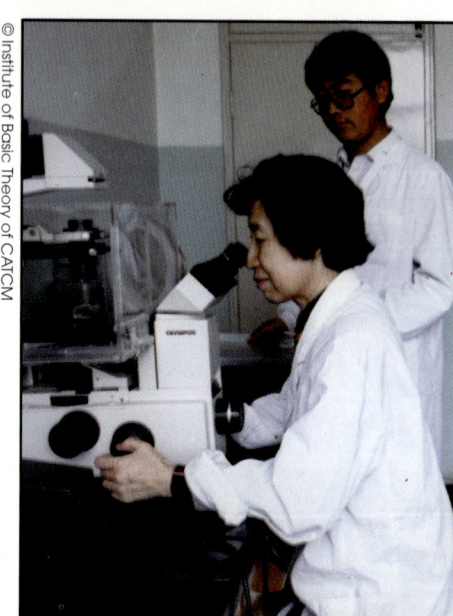

Fig.22 Guan Chongfen, director of the Immunology Department, Institute of Basic Theory, China Academy of Traditional Chinese Medicine.

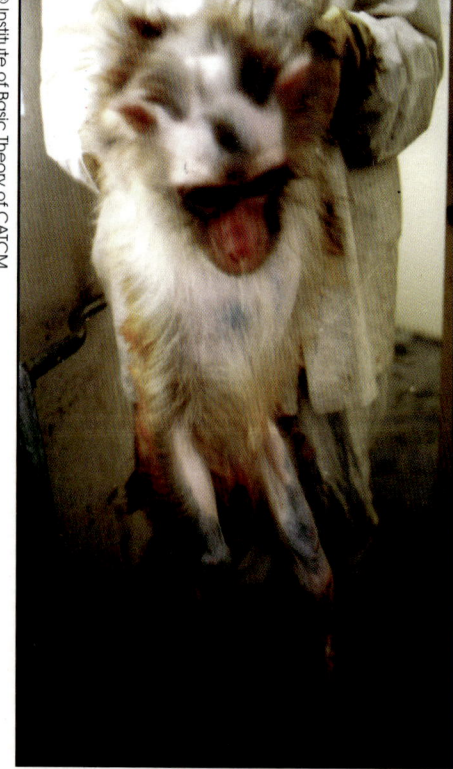

Fig.23 Simian (monkey) AIDS model infected with simian immunodeficiency virus (SIV). The animal shows symptoms of emaciation, depilation and weakness.

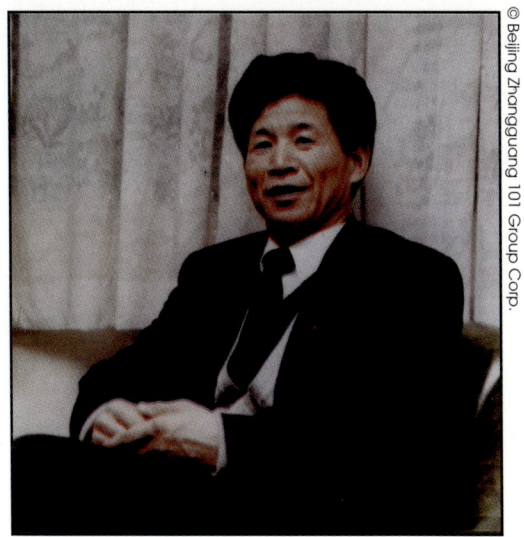

Fig.24 Zhao Zhangguang, inventor of *101* Hair Regeneration Tincture.

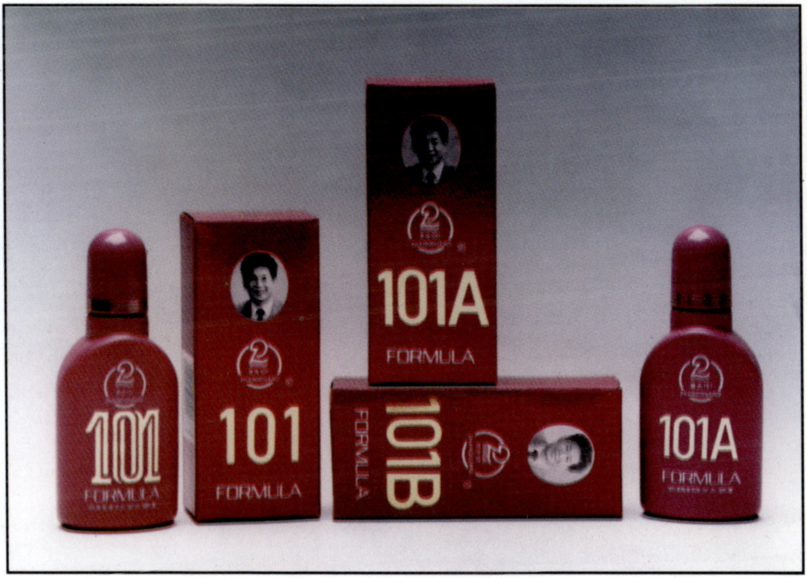

Fig.25 Packaged *101* hair regeneration products.

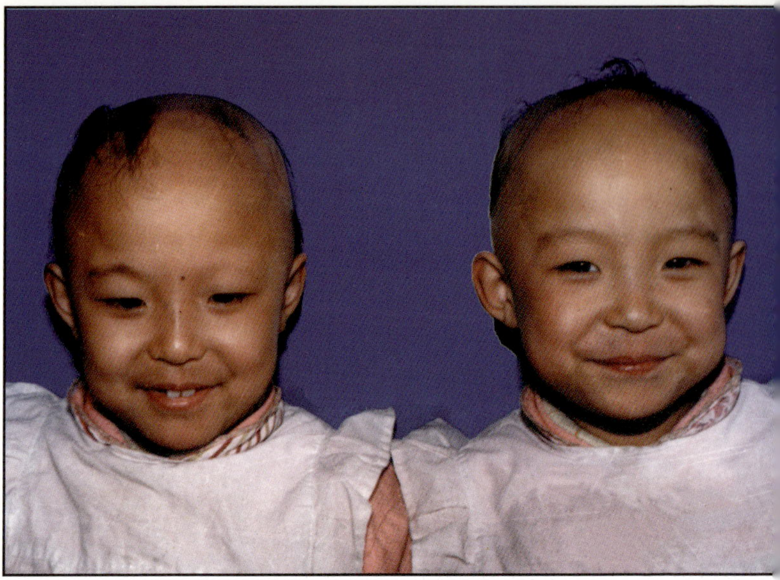

Fig.26 Twin girls before treatment. They suffered hair loss for more than three years.

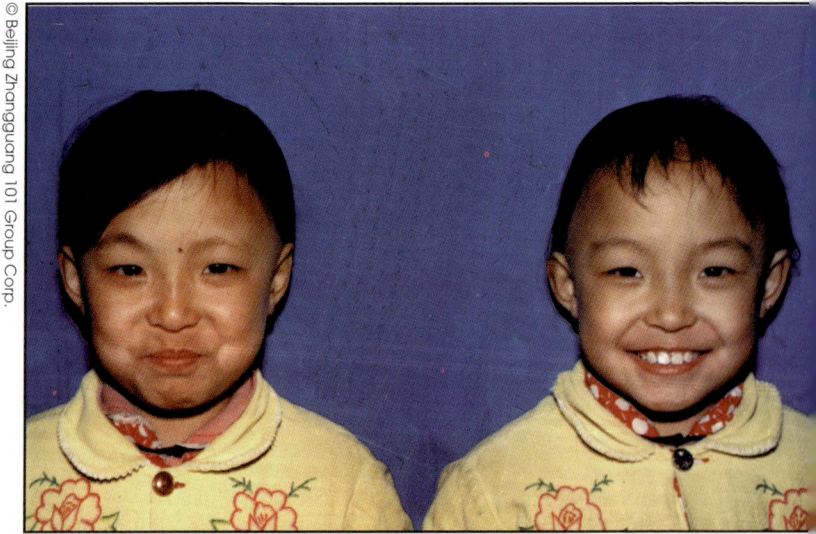

Fig.27 The twins with thick heads of hair after six months' treatment with *101* Hair Regeneration Tincture.

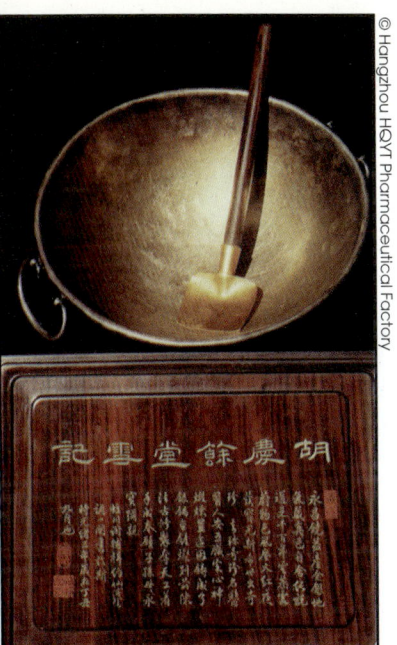
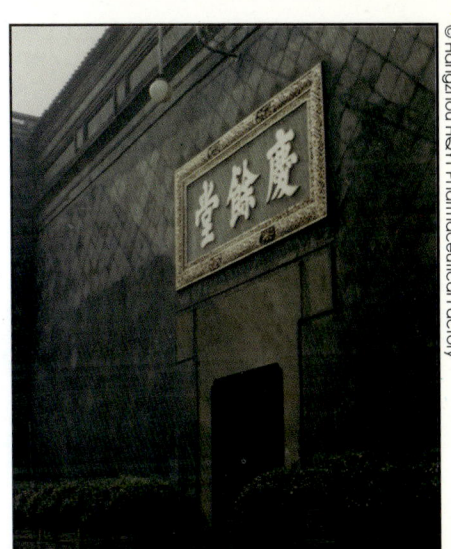

Fig.28 Gold spatula and silver pan designed and used by Hu Xueyan, founder of *Hu Qing Yu Tang*.

Fig.29 Entrance to *Hu Qing Yu Tang*.

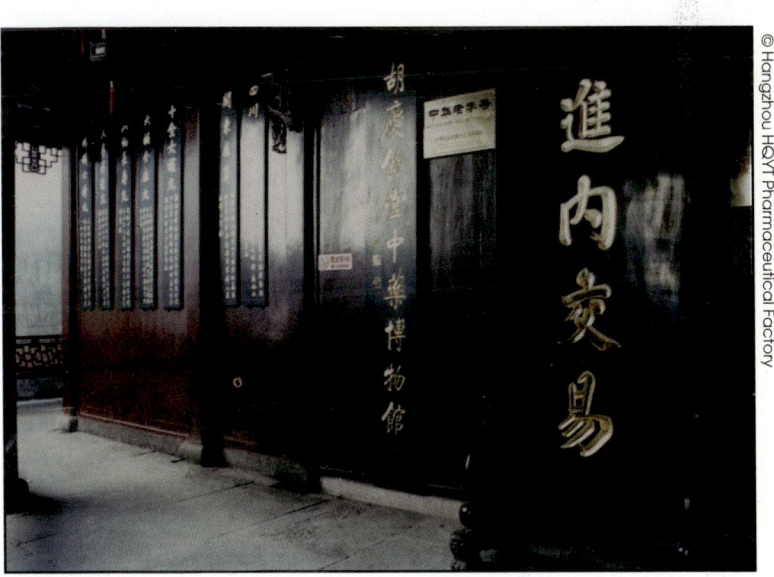

Fig.30 *Hu Qing Yu Tang* Museum of Traditional Chinese Medicines, which houses a collection of medicines and apparatus chronicling the development of the practice. The oldest exhibits display excavated medicines dating back between 3,000 and 7,000 years.

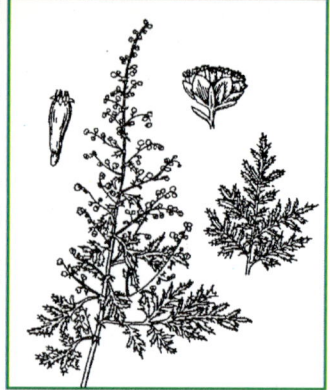

Fig.31 The medicinal herb *Qing Hao* (*Artemisia Annua Linn*).

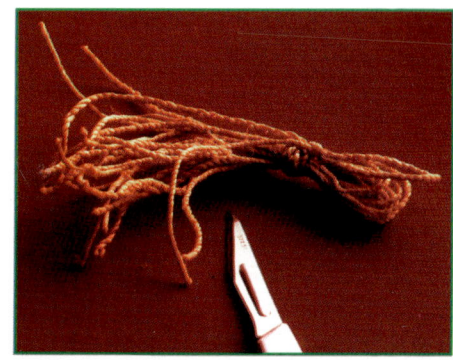

Fig.21 Medicated threads, about 0.7 mm in diameter.

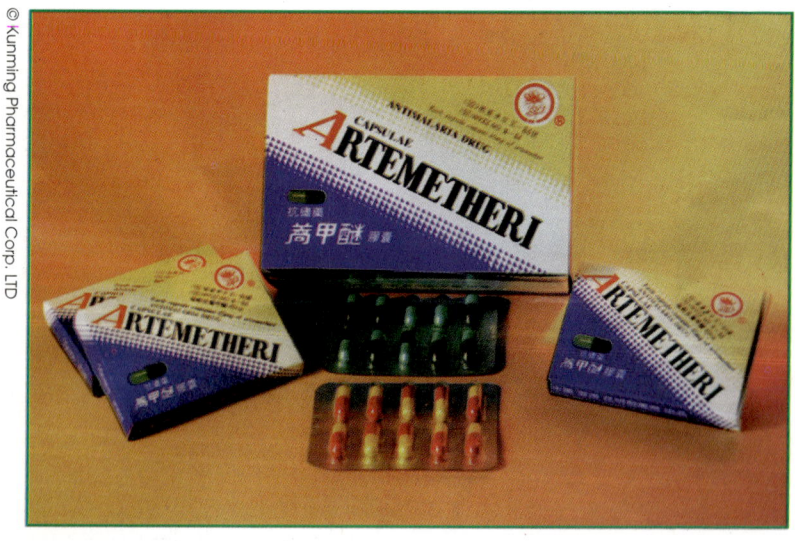

Fig.32 Packaged Artemether capsules.

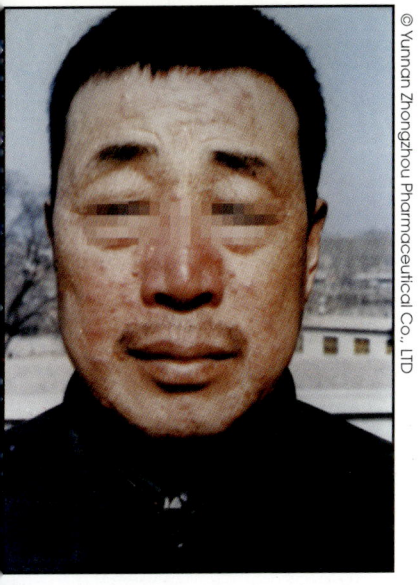

Fig.35 52-year-old acne sufferer Tao Mingyou, before treatment.

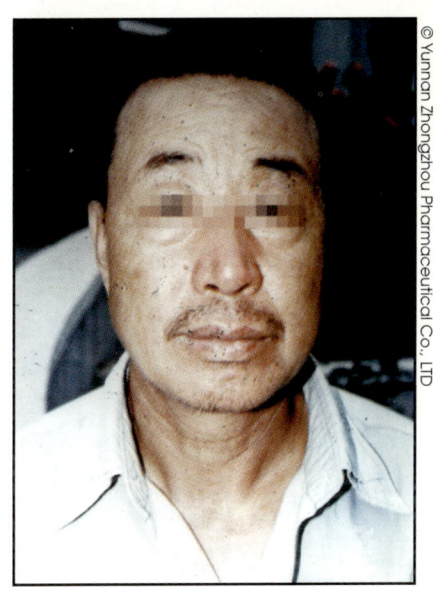

Fig.36 Two months after treatment with *Zhongzhou* Ointment, patient Tao Mingyou had a much-improved complexion.

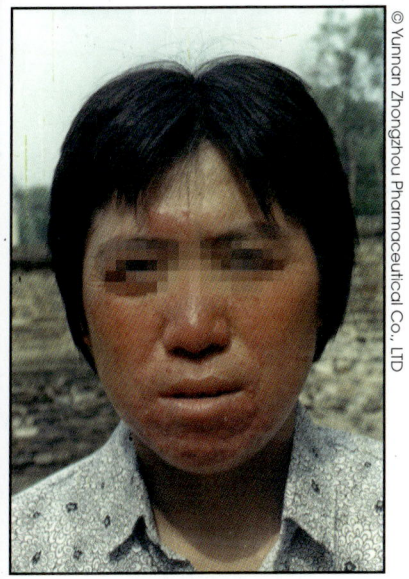

Fig.37 Acne sufferer Dang Hailing, before treatment.

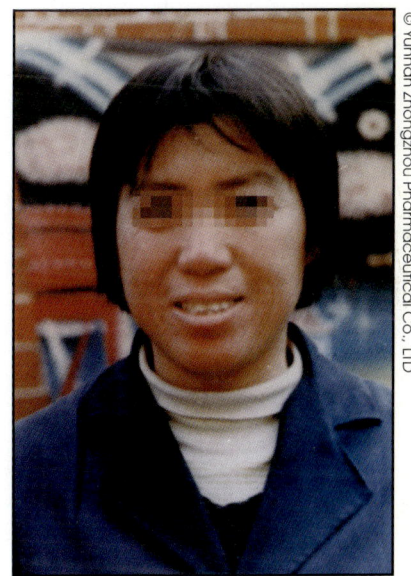

Fig.38 Dang Hailing after 72-days' treatment with *Zhongzhou* Ointment.

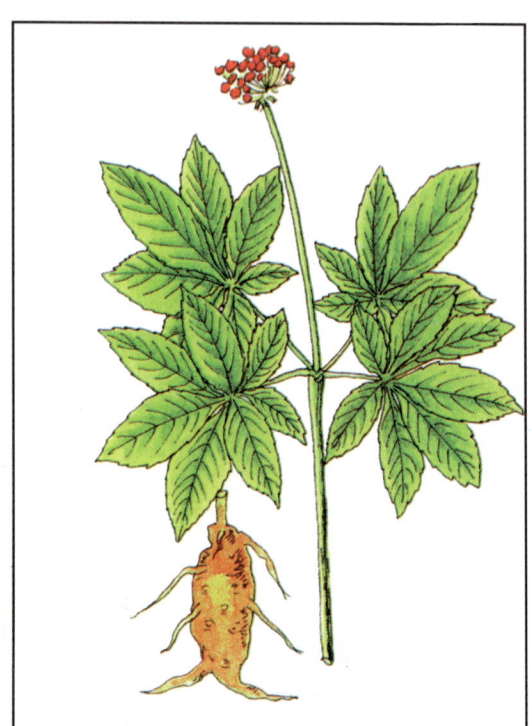

Fig.19 *Notoginseng*. The dried root of *notogingseng* comprises the main ingredient of White Medicine. It primarily functions to arrest bleeding, remove blood stasis and relieve pain.

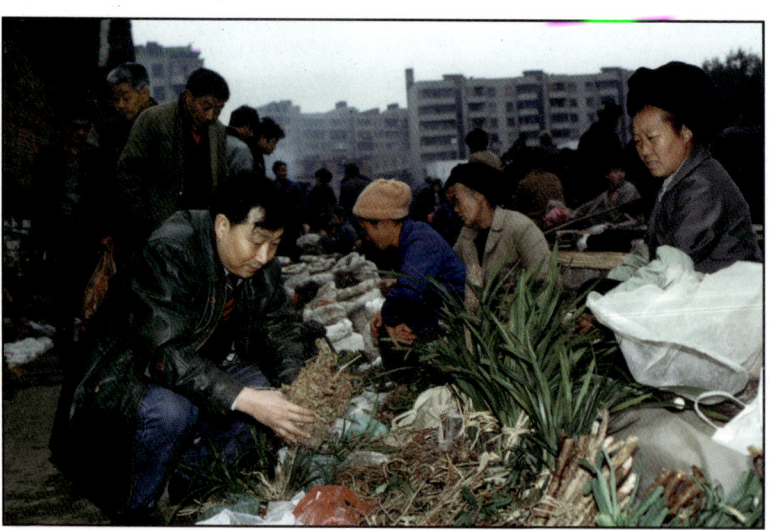

Photo by Hou Shaohua

Fig.39 Liao Hongyou examines the quality of medicinal herbs at Yangming Road medicine market in Guiyang, capital of Guizhou Province, where local people gather to sell herbs, flowers and birds.

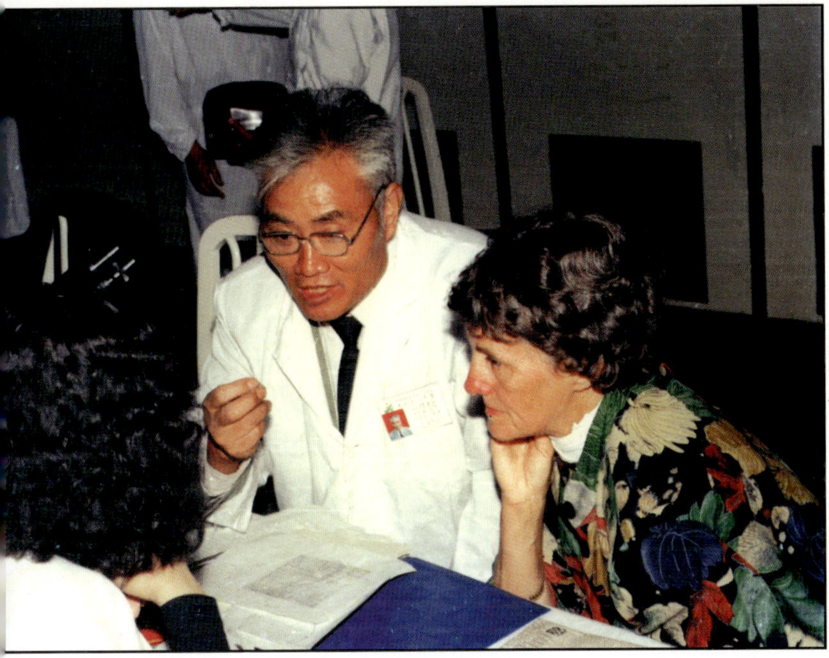

Fig.34 Zhao Zhongzhou, inventor of *Zhongzhou* Ointment, talks to foreign patients about his method for treating acne.

Photo by Wang Zhenshan

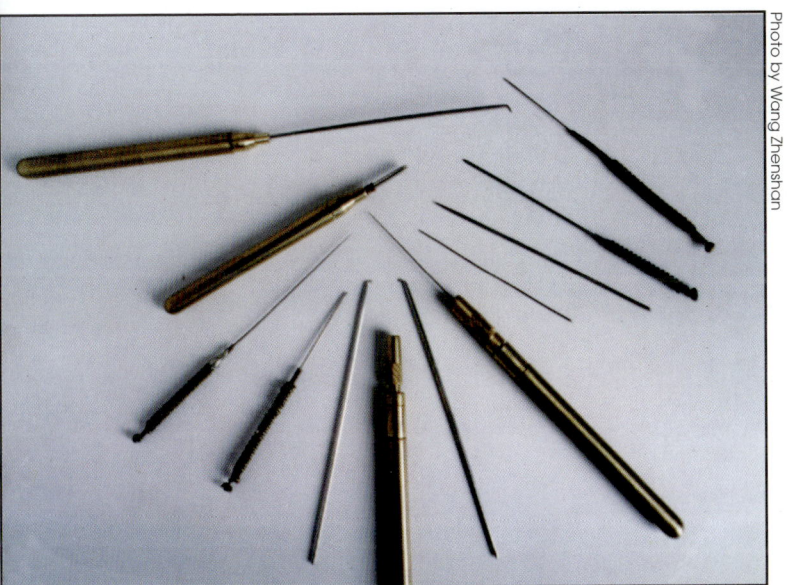

Fig.11 Fire needles made by You Fushan. The hooked needle (longest) is designed to treat spurs.

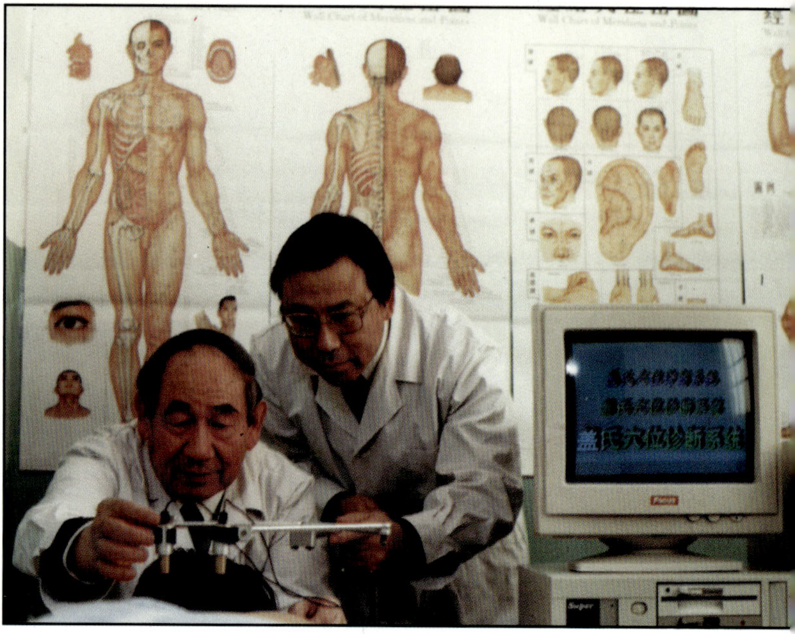

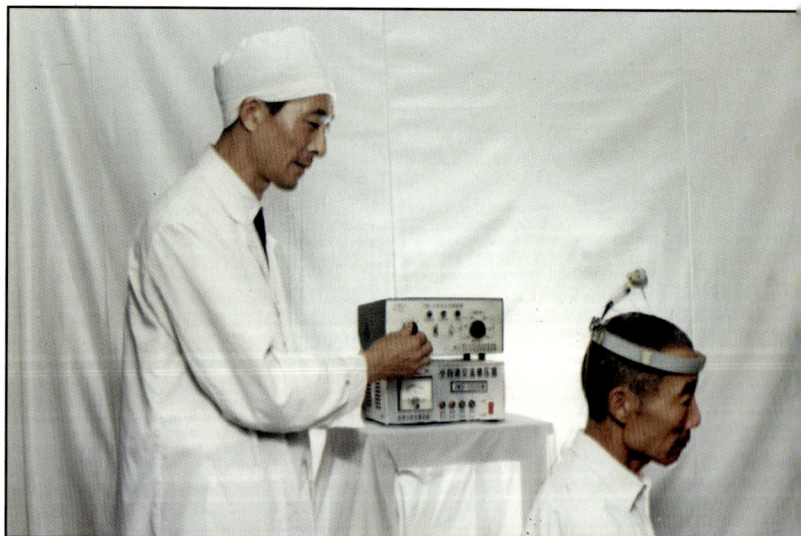

Fig.40 Father and son, Gai Guocai (left) and Gai Hua, work on the GAI Channel Points Diagnosis System.

Fig.33 Chen Daoyi uses the electric stimulator to strengthen the therapeutic effect of scalp acupuncture.

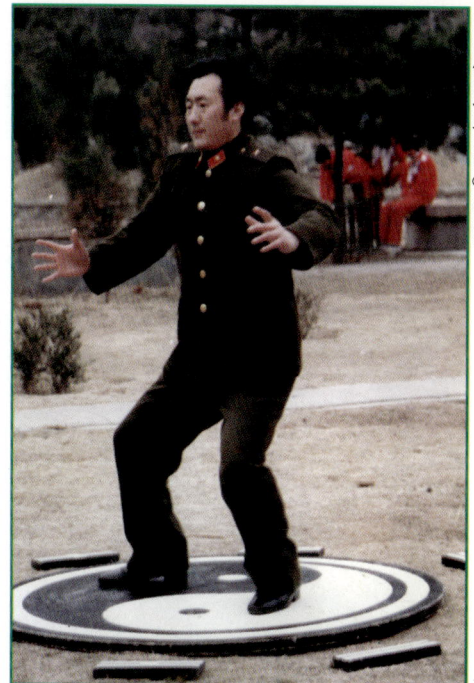

Fig.41 Wan Sujian practices a deep-breathing exercise which he named as *Bagua Xundao Gong*.

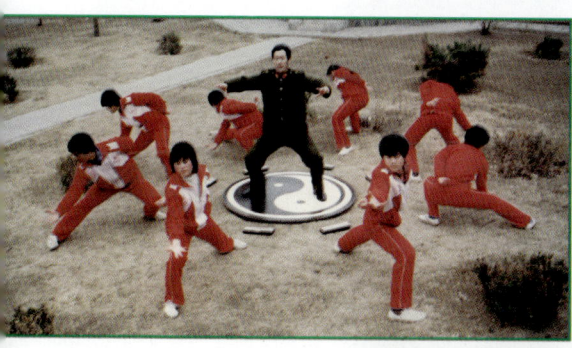

Fig.42 Wan Sujian instructs his students to invigorate their vital energy *qi* by doing *Bagua Xundao Gong*.

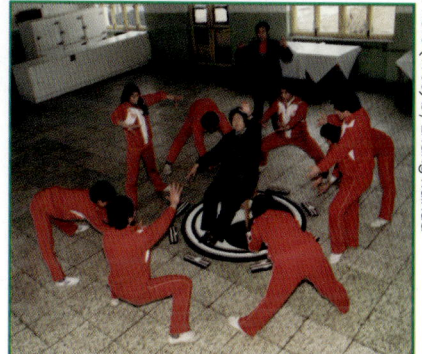

Fig.43 Wan Sujian directs his students in treating a hemiplegia sufferer (middle) from eight directions.

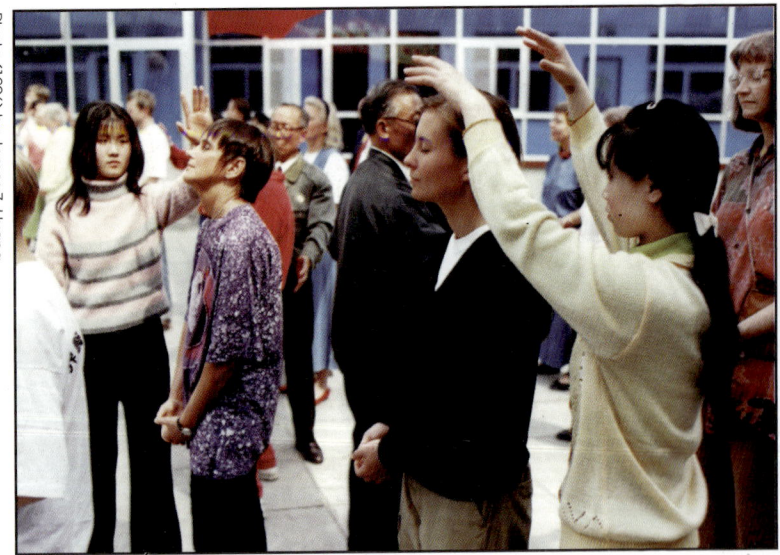

Fig.44 In September 1996, an International Medical *Qigong* Seminar was held at Wan Sujian's new hospital in Beijing. *Qigong* enthusiasts from around the world came to exchange views and skills acquired in their own medical *qigong* practices.

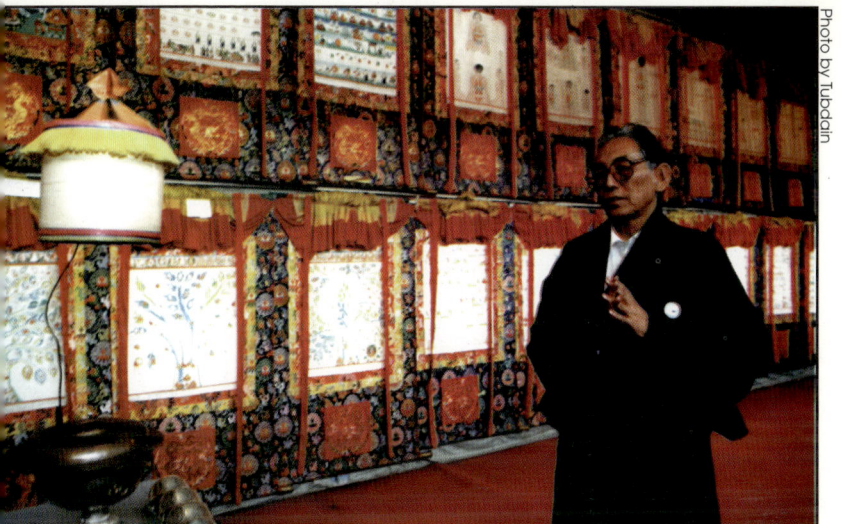

Fig.45 Jampa Tiley, a noted Tibetan medical scholar, prays in front of founders of Tibetan medicine through the ages. The background is adorned with medical *thangkas*.

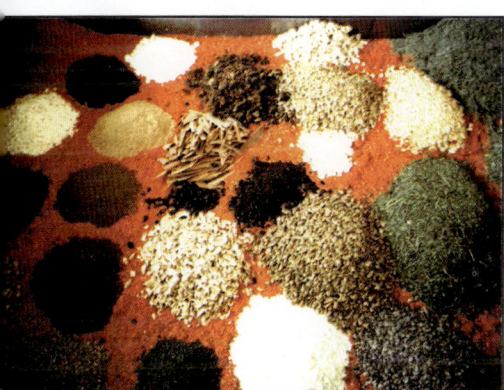

Fig.46 Rare medicinal herbs of Tibetan medicine.

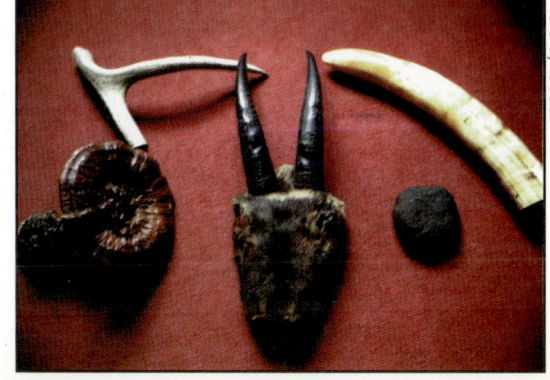

Fig.47 Plant and animal parts used in Tibetan medicine.

Photo by Tubdain

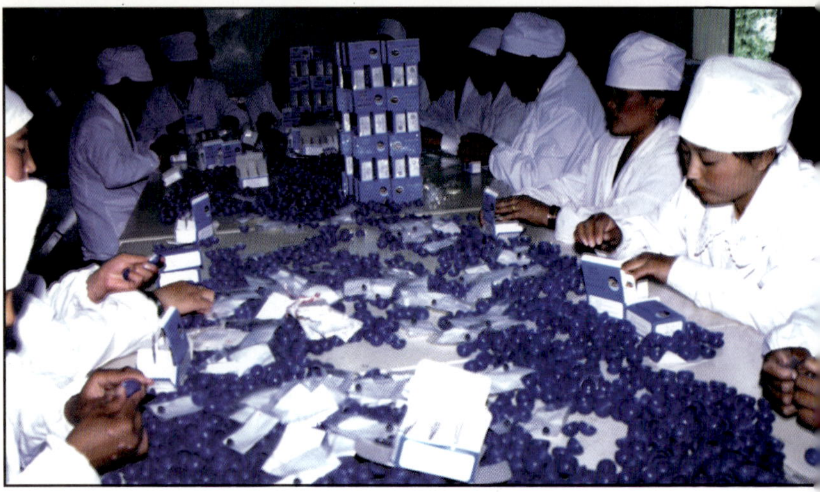

Fig.48 Medical workers of the Regional Hospital of Tibetan Medicine pack herbal drugs.

Photo by Tubdain

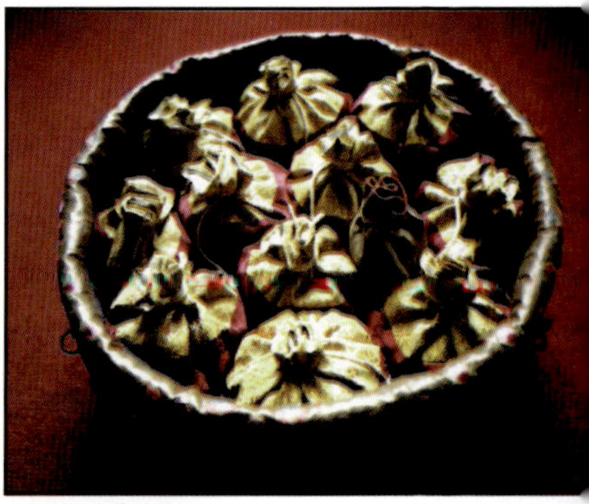

Fig.49 Tibetan medicine kit. The basket, made of yak skin, contains a dozen sheep- and deer-skin pouches, each filled with a different herbal medicine.

Photo by Tubdain

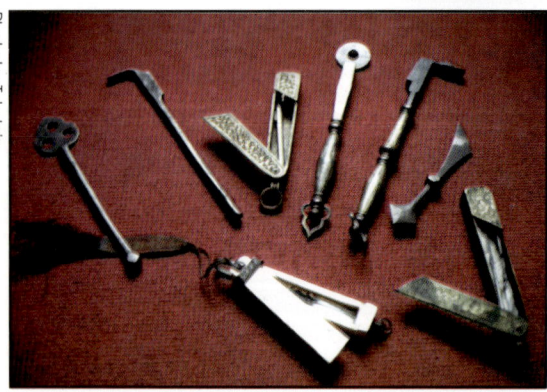

Fig.50 Medical instruments used by Tibetan medicine doctors have remained unchanged for hundreds of years.

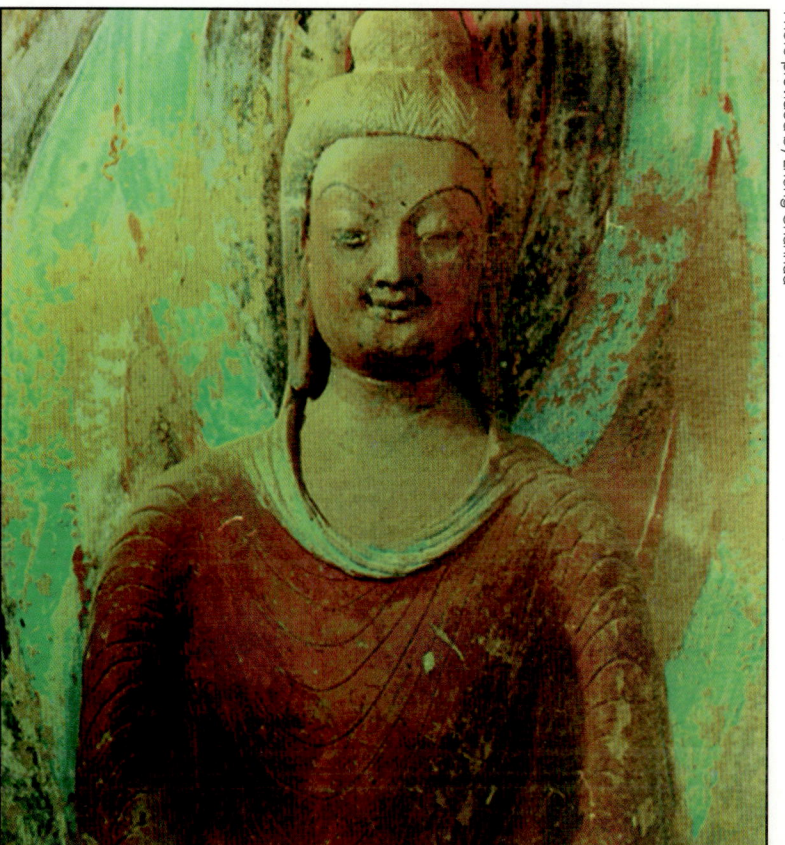

Fig.51 A painted clay figurine from the Northern Wei Dynasty Cave 259: the Buddha in the position of Zen – meditation and deep breathing.

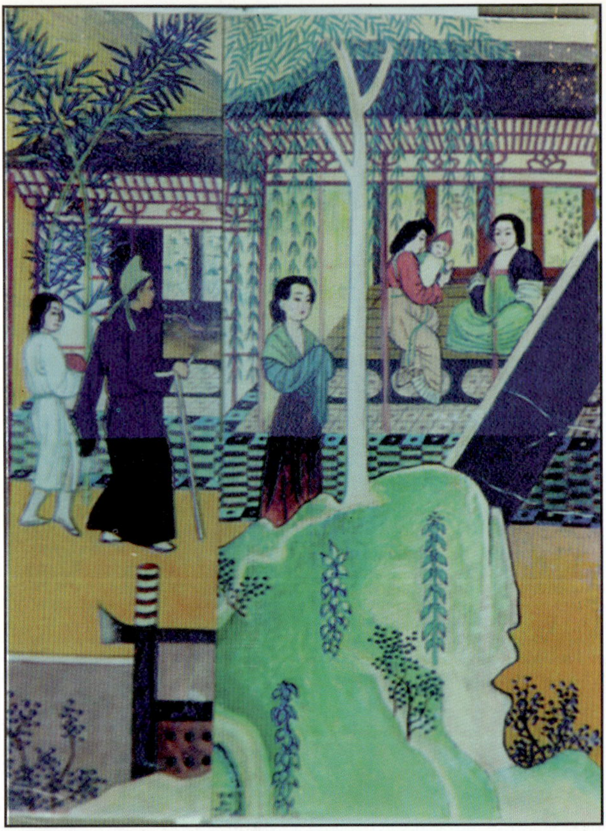

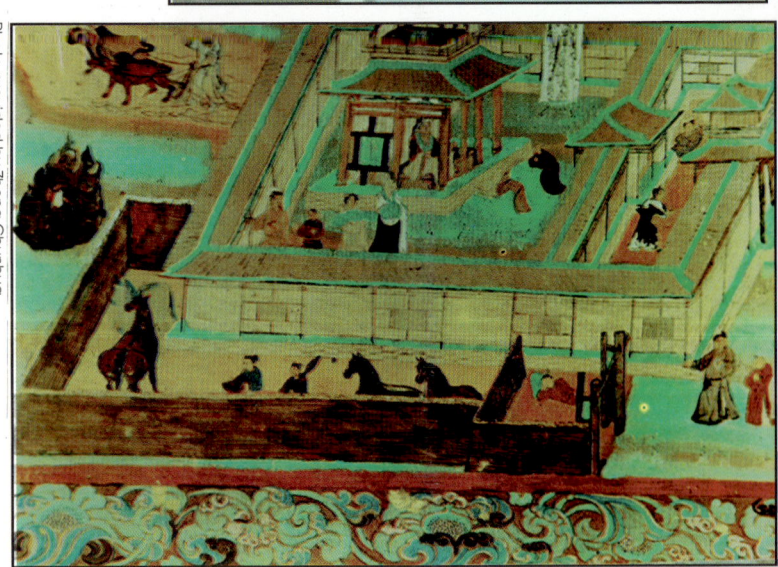

Fig.52 Artist's copy of a mural from the south wall of the Tang Cave 217: A working clinic.

Fig.53 Late-Tang mural from Cave 85 depicting the cleaning of a stable. The scene evidences the ancients' concern for environmental sanitation.

his age.

Despite repeated visits to hospitals in Guiyang, capital of southwest China's Guizhou Province, in quest for treatment to close up the old fracture, no practitioner could do the job.

Xia Wei's fortune finally turned when he was examined by a local folk doctor, Liao Hongyou.

With a little help from modern medical technology, an X-ray machine, Liao located the problem — a gaping one-centimeter wide crack in the boy's occipital bone. Then he prescribed some herbal medicine. Just three weeks later the fissure had almost closed and the boy, by and large, became normal in movement and facial appearance.

The miracle medicine, *Su Xiao Nao Fu Kang,* which translates literally as "instant brain cure," has been verified by the Guizhou provincial medical authorities as effective for treating cerebral diseases. Specifically, it is able to reduce blood viscosity, soften hardened arteries and improve blood circulation in general.

Over the past year, Doctor Liao Hongyou and his colleagues have used the medicine to treat 204 patients struck down with cerebral hemorrhages. Results were rated as "effective" in 96 percent of the cases and "markedly effective" in 71 percent. Ninety-five of his patients can now walk without assistance and not a single case of relapse has been reported from any of them.

Liao Hongyou, 51, is deputy president of the Guizhou Chinese Herbal Medicine Hospital and director of a clinic specializing in treating bone injuries, kidney and gall-stones. Experiences of his own and many others show that herbal medicine, even though regarded by some as primitive, may produce miraculous results — provided it is properly administered.

"The plant kingdom is a medicinal treasure house, though somewhat mysterious," Liao says. "It can provide effective treatment for some diseases that defy modern medicine, though it's often difficult to explain in scientific terms exactly why it works."

Indeed, Liao is known far and wide for using self-developed herbal medicines to treat cerebral vessel diseases, bone fractures, gall bladder- and kidney-stones, Meniere's syndrome, hydrophobia, scleroderma, and gout.

Like most folk doctors in China, Liao inherited his ability to concoct and administer herbal medicines.

"I began to learn from my parents when a child," he recalled. "They taught me to collect and identify medicinal herbs in the wild."

Despite his childhood fascination for cures from the forest, as a teenager he was forced to take up other work. Upon leaving higher middle school, Liao became a factory worker. "But I continued learning, spending all my spare time pouring over classic traditional Chinese medicine works."

Those classics included *Huang Di Nei Jing* (*The Yellow Emperor's Internal Classic*) from the 4th century B.C., and *Compendium of Materia Medica*, an ancient Chinese encyclopedia of pharmacy and botany by Li Shizhen (1518-1593). They are regarded as "Bibles" of traditional Chinese medicine.

Fortunately for Liao, he is a native of Guizhou Province. The Yunnan-Guizhou Plateau has an enormous assemblage of plant life with medicinal value. Moreover, the region is home to dozens of ethnic groups including the Miao, Dong, Zhuang, Yi, Hui, Buyi and Tujia. All these nationalities have developed their own ways of using local plants to treat and prevent diseases.

In most cases, these folk prescriptions and methods of treatment have been passed from generation to generation by word of mouth. And they are highly valued remedies. For example, the contents of medicinal preparations are never divulged to daughters because they marry into other families, taking secret knowledge with them.

"Man can't afford to lose these remedies," Liao says. "That's why I set for myself the task of collecting them and using them to treat patients."

One of the numerous folk prescriptions Liao has acquired is *Che Che Yao*, used for setting broken bones. He traded medical knowledge with a Yi nationality folk doctor living deep in the Wumeng Mountains, about 200 kilometers from Guiyang. "It involved a lot of bargaining," he says. "*Che Che Yao* was a family secret and I had to offer my own prescriptions for treating acute hepatitis and diarrhea in exchange."

Once obtained, Liao made a painstaking study of the preparation, and used it to improve his own "*Jiren* Bone-Setting Powder." While stopping pain, relieving inflammation and improving circulation, the powder sets bone fractures without the conventional need for bandaging and plaster. Its administration has proved effective in more than 1,000 cases with 97 percent of the patients showing complete recovery.

One such fortunate patient is Han Fengjia, an electrician at a local distillery. The 56-year old fractured his hip, ribs and legs in an horrific fall from the balcony of the fifth floor of his factory in February 1996.

After 10 oral doses of *Jiren* Bone-Setting Powder over a 10-week period his fractures had completely closed.

Wang Daxin, also from Guiyang, had a thigh bone deadened with pseudoarthrosis. Doctors practicing Western medicine diagnosed his condition incurable, even with bone transplanting.

Desperate, the patient asked Liao for help. Again the *Jiren* powder worked: two months after the patient began taking it, his leg movement was restored.

Liao's Stone Dissolver is another remarkable medicine, but this one treats internal ailments. As the name suggests, the preparation dissolves stones, in the urinary system which, in many cases, are then discharged from the body. Thousands of patients suffering from stones in various parts of the abdomen have benefited from the dissolver. It has proved effective in 97.5 percent of recorded cases.

Long Chenglan is one of them. She had multiple stones in her liver and the common bile duct, the largest in the internal duct of the liver being 1.6cm across and another in the common bile duct, 2.1cm in diameter. By the time she visited Liao, the woman, in her late 50s, resembled a walking skeleton.

But one week after taking *Liao's* Stone Dissolver, she found that her appetite was picking up. Ultrasound scans showed that stones in the common bile duct had disappeared, and the largest one in the internal duct of the liver was fighting a losing battle against the miraculous dissolver — it had been reduced to 0.8cm in diameter. A week later it was history. Now, two years on, Liao recently visited the woman in her home village and found her working on the farm, fighting fit, aged 60.

In treating Meniere's syndrome (an ear malady causing dizziness and deafness), Liao offers the patient a medicinal tea. Usually, after five to seven days' usage, the patient is cured. Of the more than 200 cases of Meniere's syndrome he has treated, the cure rate is "100 percent — no problem," Liao says.

Hydrophobia, or rabies, has also been tackled by Liao. He has treated 30 patients and cured them all. Unbelievable? Professor Lin Fangtao, a member of the World Health Organization Hydrophobia Advisory Group who lives in Wuhan, central China, investigated. He concluded that Liao's medicine was indeed truly remarkable.

Yet another astonishing concoction in Liao's medicine bag is a preparation for treating chronic cases of hard skin. A 32-year-old woman from Guiyang's suburbs had general scleroderma so badly that she couldn't bend her limbs. After conventional treatment her complaint actually worsened. But after taking Liao's medicine for ten days, her skin began to soften and she can now move around.

Liao has achieved stunning results with his herbal remedies, time after time. It seems that he can treat every ailment he tackles with success. Even the least skeptical of people could be excused for harboring some elements of doubt. But facts are facts. And his facts are recovered patients.

Folk medicine remains shrouded in mystery. The secrecy surrounding the contents of the preparations themselves adds to the mystery. But no matter how skeptical people are about its effectiveness, all folk doctors in the profession keep their mouths shut.

Liao is one of them. He refuses to divulge the ingredients of any medicine he has developed. Experience is his guarantee. "I've been allowed to practice medicine since 1966," he says.

That's 30 years of experience which speaks for itself.

FOR RELEVANT ILLUSTRATION, SEE Fig. 39.

CHAPTER 20

A BREAK FROM TRADITIONAL PATIENCE

Most Chinese doctors consider time to be the key factor in promoting the healing of fractures. Liu Haifeng is not one of them. His bone-setting powder, Sanhua Jiegu San, a ground up mixture of herbs, insects and minerals, promotes blood circulation and stimulates the growth of bone forming cells. That translates very simply into a short cut to healing breaks.

It has long been accepted by ordinary Chinese that those suffering from fractures have to undergo lengthy courses of treatment on their roads to recovery. Oft-quoted words of wisdom illustrate a belief in the absence of short cuts: "You should rest for at least 100 days if your tendons or bones are injured."

But Liu Haifeng, director of the Beijing Capital Institute of Osteopaedical Traumatology, challenges such cautious advice with his own traditional Chinese medicine (TCM) which, he claims, can get some patients back on their feet in as little as 28 days.

Ten years ago, adapting a secret recipe handed down from his ancestors, Liu prepared a fracture-setting powder to cure traumatic injuries. Long-term clinical practices have shown that the new drug has an overall effective rate of 97.6 percent. And it also boasts a 97 percent cure rate when prescribed for such injuries as new fractures, soft tissue injuries, delayed union of bones and non-union.

TCM theory places much emphasis on *qi* (or vital energy), believed to be a dynamic force having a direct bearing on blood circulation. Smooth *qi* can engender a smooth blood flow. Conversely, disturbed *qi* produces turbulence and illness. When a fracture occurs, blood flows out of its channels at the injured site, which in turn leads to blood stasis (circulation stoppage) and channel blockage. The stasis and blockage not only give pain to the patient, but also disrupt the circulation of both *qi* and blood in the internal organs of the human body. This makes fracture-setting difficult.

TCM practitioners therefore believe that, in curing traumatic injuries, patients should be prescribed preparations which promote blood circulation and remove obstruction in the channels, after taking reposition treatment.

Complying with this principle, Liu's medicine has properties to reduce swelling, alleviate pain, relax muscles and tendons and promote blood circulation.

The compound comprises more than 20 herbal, faunal and inorganic ingredients, including *Radix Notoginseng, Radix Angelicae Sinensis, Stiga Croci, Rhizoma Ligustici Chuanxiong*, ground beetles and pyrites, a brassy-yellow ferrous mineral. *Radix Notoginseng*, called *San Qi* in Chinese, is the chief component of the drug: it has the efficacy of eliminating blood stasis and reducing swelling. *Stigma Croci* and *Rhizoma Ligustici Chuanxiong* can nourish blood and relieve pain, while pyrites is believed to help set fractures.

"In preparing *Sanhua Jiegu San*, I follow the principles of Western medicine in the understanding of pathological changes and the healing process," says 38-year-old Liu Haifeng.

When a fracture happens, bleeding, inflammation and necrosis (local death of part of the living body) occur. This is followed by a restoration period of porosis, or the formation of callus, new material by which fractured bones are consolidated.

In this process, the healing progress depends on the development of tissues. If blood in the fracture site circulates well, blood clots will be absorbed by the body, and fibrous tissues will quickly develop to become bony calluses. If blood circulation is poor, the healing process will be much slower. Good blood circulation, therefore, is crucial for the rapid repair of a fracture.

"My drug brings about fracture healing by repairing tissues damaged by bleeding and inflammation: it activates blood circulation and finally promotes the formation of bony calluses," says Liu Haifeng.

Born into a TCM practitioner's family in Shuangyashan, a city in northeast China's Heilongjiang Province, Liu Haifeng followed in his father's footsteps, and beyond. "I often saw my father use a huge pot in our courtyard to decoct herbal preparations which had been known in the family for years," he recalls. "Whenever patients suffering from traumatic injuries came for treatment, he would prescribe the decoctions."

But it was an emergency situation that really sparked off Liu's interest in the effectiveness of the old family recipe. After graduating from Jilin School of Traditional Chinese Medicine, Changchun, in 1977, Liu was assigned as a medic in a local construction company. One of the workers, Li Fengchun, broke his leg after a fall. After receiving treatment from doctors, Li still felt unbearable pain.

When Liu Haifeng examined Li, he wrote a prescription for the injured worker according to his own secret recipe. Just 15 minutes after taking Liu's medicine, the worker felt his pains being alleviated. Seven days later, swellings had gone down. Twenty days later, an X-ray showed that the fracture had set.

Inspired by this remarkable initial success, Liu Haifeng embarked on research and experiments on the secret recipe. Between 1986 and 1988 he focused his research on the form — liquid or solid — of the medicine, and its dosage.

"It was quite difficult to work out the optimum dosage of the decoction — and another thing, I thought liquid forms were rather inconvenient," says Liu Haifeng. "So I chose to grind the medicinal herbs and other ingredients into powder form with pestle and mortar," he says. Regarding the amount administered, Liu experimented with various incremental doses, up to a maximum of 20 grams. He finally concluded that five-gram dosages achieved the best results.

In 1989, Liu Haifeng went to Beijing to continue research and experimentation on the drug. Under guidance from orthopedic experts and researchers from Beijing Children's Hospital, Capital Medical College and the Institute of Traditional Chinese Medicine, Liu conducted a range of comprehensive pharmacodynamic, pathological and toxicological experiments over three years.

"We used 220 dogs, 280 rabbits and 1,800 white rats in our lab work," says Liu.

With that guinea-pig experimentation satisfactorily concluded, the new drug was made available in seven of Beijing's hospitals. According to Chinese Ministry of Public Health regulations, 450 successful clinical cases must be recorded on file for a new medicine to be granted a commercial production permit. In September 1994, the ministry appointed four more hospitals at which to conduct a second round of clinical tests on the medicine.

One year later, the four hospitals submitted to the Ministry of Public Health a joint report on the effectiveness of the fracture-setting powder relating to 450 clinical cases. "This medicine can absorb hematoma (blood-related swelling) at an early stage and stimulate the increase of osteoblasts (bone-forming cells) in the periosteum (a tough fibrous membrane covering the surface of bones). Hence it promotes the early healing of fractures. Some patients who took this medicine were healed in 28 days. The total efficacious rate is 97.6 percent," stated the report.

In November 1995, the first batch of the fracture-setting powder was produced by Liu's own pharmaceutical factory based in Yingkou, in northeast China's Liaoning Province.

And while it took Liu Haifeng ten years to turn his secret recipe into a state-licensed drug, the product still had to win high regard for itself among doctors and patients.

"At first I was very skeptical — I really couldn't believe that a Chinese drug was capable of setting fractures," says Pan Shaochuan, orthopedic surgeon and director of the surgical department of Beijing Children's Hospital.

Pan changed his view when he witnessed the drug's performance in curing children's congenital pseudoarthrosis of the shinbone, a condition caused by neurofibroma (tumor on the nerve tissues).

Teenager Guo Lingmin was suffering from the disease and went to Beijing Children's Hospital for treatment. Doctors treated her in the conventional way by fixing her shin with a "fixator" (an adjustable, rather cumbersome device to promote healing of a shin fracture). But the fracture did not heal, even after prolonged treatment. Desperate for a breakthrough, doctors resorted to Liu Haifeng's fracture-setting drug. Just 45 days later the fracture had healed.

"On the precedent of Guo Lingmin's case, we've treated similar problems the same way," says director Pan.

Gao Zhanxiang, formerly Vice-Minister of Culture, also benefited from the drug. In 1994, Gao had a fracture of the thigh bone. And because his condition was complicated by diabetes and osteoporosis, he was regarded as unfit for surgery. The fracture-setting powder was the only option. Twenty-eight days after commencing its administration, his fracture had healed.

"When I went to Hong Kong, I found that a friend was also suffering from a similar thigh injury. After experiencing various kinds of treatment for six months, his fracture still refused to heal," says Gao Zhanxiang. "So I gave him a box of Liu's powder and within six weeks he was cured."

To date, Liu Haifeng has revealed 18 medicinal ingredients of his recipe — but he keeps the exact method of its preparation and an additional secret material, a guiding drug that can direct drugs to act on a certain channel or site, a closely-guarded secret.

Five grams of the fracture-setting powder is packed into a sachet, with 28 sachets being packed into one carton. One course of treatment lasts 14 days, during which the drug is taken orally twice a day, one sachet each time. Usually patients are recommended two courses.

"At US$168, the powder is expensive for ordinary Chinese," admits Liu Haifeng, "but it enjoys a quite good market because it's known to work," he says. So far, his company has set up a sales network in 16 provinces across China.

"We aim to extend our network to all provinces and regions eventually," says an ambitious Liu. "At the same time, I want to continue my research on the growth of bone cells in the human body as my effort to produce a cure for the development of porous structures in the bones of the elderly."

CHAPTER 21

FOR THE HEALTH OF NEWBORN BABIES

Spina bifida, causing babies to be physically and mentally retarded for life, affects up to 100,000 newborns a year in China. Yet this disabling disease is actually caused by a simple deficiency of a B-complex vitamin — folic acid — during pregnancy. Heading a Sino-US team searching for a solution to the deficiency, Li Zhu of Beijing Medical University has developed a dietary supplement pill, Scrianen, which can reduce the incidence of neural tube defect (NTD) births by 80 percent.

Every six minutes, a baby with neural tube defects (NTDs) is born in China. He or she may have no skull, or have incomplete brain tissues. His or her spine may be deformed with the spinal cord protruding.

In China only ten percent of NTD babies can survive. If they do, they will be afflicted with spina bifida, handicapped for life, suffering from leg paralysis, incontinence, skin diseases and infections of the urinary system. Anencephalic infants — those with all or the majority of their brains missing — die soon after birth.

Zuo Lijuan's dearest wish is to see blue sky and green fields, and go to school like the other children in her village. She is 12 and lives alone in a small, dark and dingy cottage in a corner of a courtyard of

Yuanshi County, Hebei Province. Born with spina bifida, the poor girl can only move with the support of a stool used in walking-stick fashion.

Zuo's parents spent a large sum of money on several operations for her, but the surgery failed to improve her condition.

As the most common and most severe birth defect both in China and in the world, NTDs occur in about 400,000 infants every year. Some 80,000-100,000 of them occur in China.

While the NTD birth rate is 0.3-2.1 per thousand in 20 or more foreign countries, China's rate is 2.3-2.8 per thousand. In some northern parts of the country the incidence is as high as 10 per thousand, or one percent, ten times more serious than in many developed countries.

"No wonder China's dubbed the Himalayas of NTDs — it's such a tragedy," says Professor Li Zhu, 48, of Beijing Medical University (BMU).

If an expectant mother eventually loses her baby, she will be psychologically traumatized as well as having lost a considerable sum of money spent on nutritious food during her pregnancy. She may also have taken leave from work – an economic loss for society. Moreover, she may not be able to return and perform her duties effectively as a result of post natal depression.

If an NTD birth occurs, parents are traumatized and face high charges for surgery on their disabled child, at least 5000 yuan (US$600) which may be as much as a year's earnings for an average worker. Furthermore, the child may require constant care and attention, necessitating one of the parents to quit their job, which would inevitably effect the family budget for years to come.

Yet most NTD births can be prevented, says Prof. Li, who has been cooperating, on behalf of the BMU-based National Center for Maternal and Infant Health (NCMIH), with the United States Center for Disease Control and Prevention (CDC), to combat NTDs.

Since Li and his colleagues detected and reported the high occurrence of NTDs in China in 1983, they have conducted lengthy research into finding a way to reduce its incidence.

Li is the principal investigator on the US-China Collaborative Project for NTDs Prevention. With a budget of US$20 million, the project, from 1991 to 1997, is the biggest medical cooperative research project between the two countries.

Li and his colleagues carried out pilot research in two counties of Hebei Province between 1991 and 1993. They made tests on 1,000 women each year who planned to have children.

Dividing the women into three groups, the doctors requested one group to take vitamins which contained folic acid. Their dosages were daily, from one month before the pregnancy until they were three months' pregnant.

The second group took folic acid only, also for the same four-month period. The third took no vitamin supplements at all..

To ensure accuracy, local doctors were employed to deliver one pill in person to each woman every day, and they were instructed to watch the women take their pills.

Li and his colleagues found that those who took folic acid lowered their risk of an NTD birth by more than 70 percent.

Li concluded that a pregnant woman's folic acid deficiency in the pre-conception month and early stage of pregnancy greatly increased the risk of her giving birth to a NTD baby.

Additionally, Li confirmed his former opinion that the NTD-incidence in North China is higher than that in South China; is higher in rural areas than in urban ones; and more commonly afflicts women whose pregnancies span winter and spring months as opposed to those who experience pregnancy during summer and fall seasons.

In fact Li first began to have such theories in 1987 when he participated in a program on nationwide birth defects surveillance.

Folic acid-rich foods include lean meat, liver and kidney, fish, eggs, green vegetables such as spinach, beans and bean products, edible wild herbs like amaranth, and fruits such as oranges and strawberries.

"Women in the city eat more vegetables than those in the countryside. The latter, who may plant vegetables, actually sell most of them. And they eat cheaper foods, rarely eating liver or fish. Another thing, fewer vegetables are available in winter and spring, so women whose pregnancies start in these seasons tend to take in less needed nourishment than those in summer and fall.

"South China has a wider variety of green vegetables than the north, where cabbage and potatoes are the main foods all through the long, cold winters. Also, on average, people in North China are less well-off than those in the south, which means they eat fewer expensive foods such as fish, eggs and liver," Li says.

Li points out that the highest incidences of NTD births occur in North China's Inner Mongolia, Heilongjiang, Shandong, Jilin, Shaanxi, Henan, Hebei and Shanxi provinces. All are north of the Yangtze River, China's longest river, which bisects the country into what is regarded as the north and south.

Li's findings coincide with the one discovered many years ago in the international medical world: that a pregnant woman with a low income and poor education, with a low standard of living, and undernourished, faces the biggest risk of experiencing an NTD birth.

Since 1993, Li and his colleagues have carried out research in 30 counties of Shanxi, Hebei, Jiangsu and Zhejiang provinces. The first two represented the area with a high incidence (the north), while the latter two represented low-incidence provinces of the south.

"Scheduled to be completed in 1997, the research is an important part of the Sino-American cooperative project," Li says. "Nearly 150,000 newly-wed women and other women who plan to get pregnant have been involved in our program and taken folic acid supplements," Li says. "By the first half of 1995, my colleagues and I formally reached a conclusion that more than 70 percent of the NTD births can be prevented if the women take folic acid supplements on a daily basis from at least one month ahead of their planned pregnancy until the end of the third month of their pregnancy."

Li's conclusion was identical to that of researchers working in the United Kingdom and Hungary.

To combat the deficiency, Li and his colleagues developed *Scrianen* to reduce the risk of NTDs. Folic acid is the major ingredient.

"The woman who intends to get pregnant is required to take one pill a day for four months. Each pill is 0.4mg," Li says.

An essential substance for the human body, folic acid is commonly deficient in Chinese women, Li says, "probably because our traditional cooking methods damage much of the nutrient and most Chinese people eat little food which contains folic acid."

Each woman needs 0.17mg of folic acid every day, Li says. The World Health Organization (WHO) suggests that a pregnant woman takes 0.4mg daily, twice the recommended daily requirement for non-pregnant women.

"Vitamins are indispensable to both the expectant mother and fetus — folic acid is essential to the anabolism of the human body and is used for synthesizing DNA," Li says.

Lack of folic acid hampers the development and maturing of red blood cells. As a result, it may lead to megaloblast anemia, which causes *abruptio placenta* and hypertension during pregnancy.

"What is more critical," Li says, "deficiency will cause defects in neural tube development of the fetus."

Li explains that embryo development begins with the cell split of the zygote. The latter will develop into a neural plate. By the end of the eighth week of pregnancy, the plate will grow into a neural tube. For the rest of the gestation, the head of the neural tube will evolve into the brain, while the end of the tube will become the spinal cord.

"That's why the NTD babies are either anencephalic or handicapped by spina bifida," Li says.

A woman farmer from Fengrun County, Hebei Province, gave birth to a pretty girl with spina bifida in September, 1992. Only a few days later the baby died of fever due to infected meningomyelocele.

Following the advice of doctors from the county's Women and Children Healthcare Center, the mother took *Scrianen* for four months starting from the end of 1992. In January 1994, she gave birth to a healthy girl. The whole family was overjoyed.

"Prevention is the best way to lower the incidence of NTD births," Li says. "Chinese people are used to eating cooked dishes, rather than raw foods. The cooking itself, including stir-frying and even frying without stirring, destroys most of the folic acid in the food. But it is not easy at all to change ideas about traditional cookery."

Li observes that the amount of food one can eat every day is quite limited. And most of the food which contains folic acid is expensive to many ordinary Chinese. Therefore it is impractical in China to dietarily supplement folic acid to the human body.

"In the United States," Li says, "scientists are trying to develop a flour fortified with folic acid. But this would not be suitable in China, for the people's dietary habits vary greatly from one place to another; it is hard to find one kind of food which all the people eat frequently. And farmers are often self-sufficient; they just eat what they grow."

In the north, flour-based staples are preferred, such as noodles and steamed bread, while in the south rice is the favorite.

"Another problem is that it will take a large amount of manpower, material resources and money to develop folic acid-fortified food."

However, taking a pill supplement such as *Scrianen* is an easy way, Li says, and it is inexpensive.

Additionally, *Scrianen* can help lower the risk of anemia and miscarriage, ease uncomfortable reactions such as morning sickness during the early stage of pregnancy, and stimulate fetal growth.

Li also believes that *Scrianen* also helps prevent the incidence of harelip cleft palate and congenital heart disease.

Graduating in 1970 from the Beijing Medical College, now BMU,

Li worked in Pingliang Prefecture in northwest China's Gansu Province until the late 1970s.

In 1981, he finished his postgraduate study at the Beijing Medical College and joined the teaching staff, focusing in particular on how women can bear and rear healthier children.

Since the Ministry of Public Health approved Li and his colleagues' application to cooperate with the American CDC to study NTDs in 1984, Li has visited the U.S. many times to facilitate the cooperation.

On September 30, 1990, US Congress approved the NTDs prevention project that was to be carried out by the two countries' scientists.

Six years later, in fall 1995, the Chinese Ministry of Public Health declared its intention to spread the project's research results concerning folic acid supplements.

"Although scientists from ten countries have advised that pregnant women should take folic acid supplements, China is the only country whose government has actually initiated the implementation. China is now leading the field of NTD research and prevention," Li says.

Smallpox vaccinations were not used worldwide until the 1960s — one century after the invention of the vaccine. "Therefore it is really significant for the Chinese government to call on the country's women to take folic acid supplements immediately after we made the finding and advised them of it — remember that about 25 million Chinese women get pregnant every year," Li says.

The Ministry of Public Health requests that, by the end of 1998, the research findings would be known throughout the whole country; and that by 2000, at least 80 percent of newly-wedded women and women intending to get pregnant should take *Scrianen*.

"Our target is to bring down the incidence by 50 percent, that is, to reduce it to 40,000-50,000 NTD births every year," Li says.

So far, both the American and Chinese sides are satisfied with the cooperation.

Peng Ruicong, Chinese chairman of the project, says: "With the Americans providing advanced technology and equipment for data collection and processing, and China arranging a large and well-organized population of participants for a long series of careful experiments on an extensive scale, the cooperation has yielded fruitful results which will benefit both nations, and all mankind."

Peng, 73, a former chairman of the BMU Board, appreciates Li's sensitiveness in grasping the opportunity.

"Since the early 1980s, Li has been playing an active role in promoting the Sino-American cooperation. He urged the CDC to set up an advanced computer network in China. If that was available, even today a doctor from a small county who is involved in our project could quickly find certain CDC data from the computer at any time."

Although the NTD study is successful, Li is not content. He wants to foster more cooperation to focus on other deformity-related subjects.

CHAPTER 22

DETECTING SIGNALS OF DISTRESS FROM TUMORS

The traditional image of Chinese medicine is shattered by one of its most recent technological innovations: the GAI tumor detector. However, the high-tech machine does work on traditional principles, and can be likened to an ultra-sensitive pair of doctor's hands. Its sensors detect abnormal bioelectrical signals emitted by tumors and passed along the meridian system of channels and collaterals, which are then picked up via acupoints on the body's surface. By translating the signals into digital and graphical information and comparing them with norms, the GAI detector can help doctors pinpoint early stage cancers, and their nature.

Zhang Song, a 41-year-old doctor at the Beijing Railway General Hospital, didn't expect that the disease which had tortured her and puzzled many American doctors for two years could be so easily detected by a machine back in her home town.

Two years ago, Zhang was sent to work at a hospital in the United States on an exchange program. One day, she felt a sudden pain in her lower stomach. At first she dismissed it as mere indigestion. But the pain grew stronger and became more regular. Towards the end of her stay in the U.S., Zhang was consulting doctors and receiving all kinds of check-ups. But no clear diagnosis could be made.

In February, 1995, Zhang Song returned home in the hope of finding out what was wrong with her stomach. To her astonishment, in only 20 minutes, a machine was able to give its operator enough information to allow him to diagnose her problem: carcinoma of the uterus. Surgery later proved there was a malignant tumor in Zhang's womb.

"Thanks to the exact diagnosis with the aid of the machine, the tumor was identified and removed at a relatively early stage," says Zhang. "Cancer isn't fatal if it's caught early enough."

It was for this very reason that Gai Guocai, a retired army doctor in Beijing, has built a machine that can detect nearly 40 kinds of tumors, including 17 kinds of malignant ones, even before the patient feels any pain or discomfort. Called the GAI tumor detector, the machine has proved 96 percent accurate in diagnosing malignant tumors and 70 percent accurate for benign ones.

"The detector works on the principles of both traditional Chinese medicine (TCM) and Western medicine," says the 70-year-old doctor. "To be exact, it makes a Western medical diagnosis based on TCM principles," he says.

Dr. Gai developed his detector on the basis of TCM which theorizes that problems in any of the internal organs, including the heart, liver, spleen, lungs, kidneys, stomach, gall, intestines and bladder, though out of sight, signal their abnormalities to the body's surface through channel acupoints.

"When a certain internal organ is abnormal (diseased), its corresponding channel points will transmit abnormal bioelectrical signals," Gai says. "I worked to build a machine that could receive and analyze such signals and transform them into computer graphics and figures."

A comprehensive analysis of the information, including a comparison of the abnormal signals with normal or expected ones, can give the doctor enough information to identify the type — malignant or benign — and stage of cancer, and its primary and secondary focus, he adds.

A Western medicine major, Gai graduated from North China Medical University in the early 1950s and began to learn acupuncture in 1956. Then he became director of the physiotherapy department of Hospital No.304 of the Chinese People's Liberation Army.

His knowledge of acupuncture and practice in the physiotherapy department helped Gai in the development of his detector. As patients came to his department by referral from the outpatient department, Gai usually knew which acupoints he needed to needle during treatment.

"Generally I felt and pressed the points with my finger tips before inserting the needle," he says. "Gradually I found that when my needle was inserted into the sore points, the patient would respond strongly — that signifies a good, strong effect. But at other points the response might be less strong, indicating a less-than-ideal effect."

That led him to realize the relationship between channel points and diseases and go on to establish the method of diagnosing diseases by receiving and comparing bioelectrical signals from these points. By the end of 1976, he had established point compositions for diagnosing 158 common diseases. His academic works on these findings have been well accepted in medical circles in China and abroad.

Yet Gai didn't stop at those achievements. He wanted to harness his method to combat perhaps the human body's worst enemy — cancer.

However, none of the 361 pairs of acupoints developed in the long history of TCM practice are ideal sites for needle insertion to identify or treat carcinogenic troubles. The doctor started work to identify such cancer-detecting channel points in 1976.

He examined hundreds of cancer patients from head to toe, altogether feeling and pressing 80,000 pair-times of channel points on 1,700 confirmed tumor patients before finally locating two new pairs of points, on the thighs, in 1978. He named them *Xin Daxi Xue* (new thigh points) and *Xin Neixi Xue* (new inside thigh points) respectively. The former points are for diagnosing malignant tumors and the latter for benign ones.

He first tried out his point diagnostic technique in a mass experiment, in 1979, on patients in Macheng, Hubei Province, a county with a high incidence of esophagus cancer. He and a medical team worked separately on the same 16,553 people, all above the age of 30, with the team using X-ray machines but Gai only using his fingers.

On completion of the survey, Gai had detected 11 cancer cases, two more than the X-ray method. Follow-up examinations proved that Gai was totally correct in diagnosing cancer in the two patients for which the X-ray machine had failed to detect.

"For centuries, channel points had been used as points for acupuncture to cure diseases only," said Wang Xuetai, former president of the World Federation of Acupuncture and Moxibustion Societies. "Gai Guocai is a pioneer in using them for diagnostic purposes. He has formulated a unique diagnostic theory on the basis of the theory of channels and collaterals and in doing so has revolutionized the diagnostic method of traditional Chinese medicine."

Despite such high praise, Gai knew it would be difficult for his method to be adopted by other practitioners because it depended largely on personal experience. He knew he needed to popularize it if it were ever to become a widely accepted method of early-stage tumor detection. A machine was what he had in mind: it needed to have sensors more sensitive than fingertips in receiving bioelectrical signals from the malignant or benign tumor.

Beginning in 1980 Gai worked to develop such a tumor detector. Over the ensuing 11-year period up to 1991 he built and improved upon five GAI machines. "The fifth generation GAI, of course, is the most advanced," says Gai Guocai, "because it can detect both the nature and location of the tumor."

The machine is convenient to use. Usually the patient lies down on his or her stomach while holding a metal probe in one hand, for circuit connecting and signal transmission. Then the doctor rolls a pen-like probe along the patient's thighs to locate two pairs of channel points — *Xin Daxi Xue* and *Xin Neixi Xue*. The machine emits a ringing signal when the correct point is located, allowing the doctor to mark it. Next, the doctor fixes a pair of sensors on each pair of the located points. Meanwhile, the sensors pick up and transmit bioelectrical signals which are transformed into graphical and digital forms on a monitor: from this the doctor can tell if there is a tumor and if so, its nature.

If a tumor is identified, the doctor uses the probes to check other points on the body to discover exactly where the tumor is located. The whole investigative process takes no more than 20 minutes.

During a clinical test at the People's Hospital in Beijing in 1992, Doctor Gai was asked to find tumor patients among 160 people with his detector. He was not provided with any of their medical histories.

The result was encouraging. The machine was 100 percent accurate in assisting Doctor Gai detect which people had tumors and where they were located. He was 87 percent accurate in detecting the nature of the tumors.

A further clinical test, on 246 people at the Beijing Railway General Hospital, showed that Doctor Gai's machine was 97 percent accurate

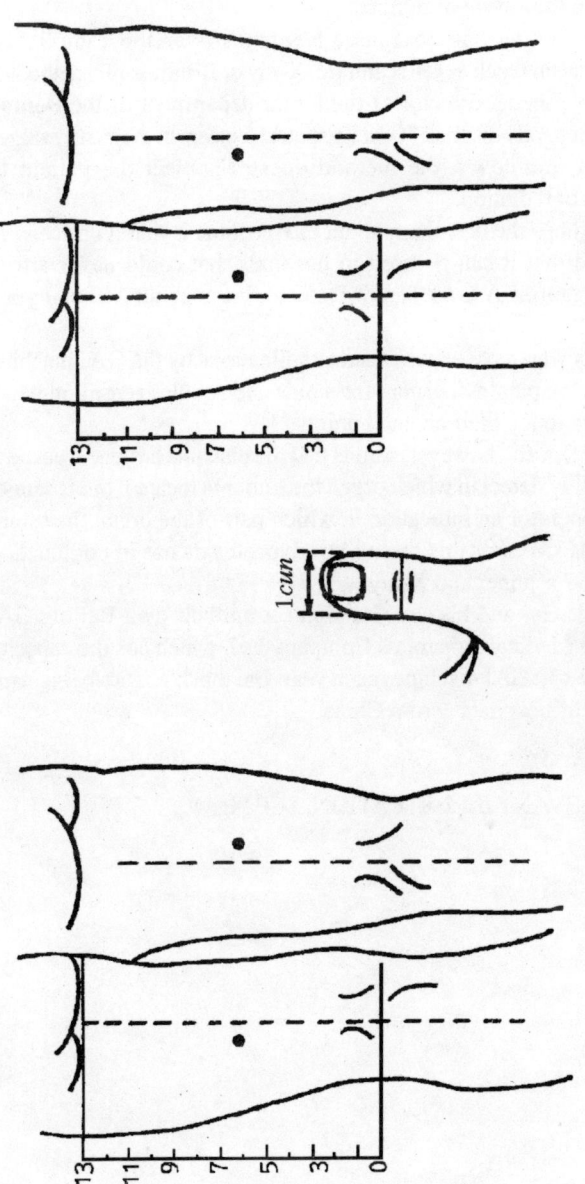

"Thumb cun," a corresponding unit of length based on the patient being treated, and used by the practitioner for locating acupoints.

Diagrams of the two pairs of points discovered by Gai Guocai — *Xin Daxi Xue* (new thigh points, left) and *Xin Neixi Xue*, (new inside thigh points, right).

in diagnosing, 96 percent in locating and 89 percent correct in identifying the nature of tumors.

"The machine has obvious advantages over the established detecting means such as CT scanning, X-ray or B-ultrasonic methods," said Du Weisheng, director of the tumor department of the Beijing Railway General Hospital. "GAI can detect cancers in their early stages of growth; moreover, the method doesn't subject the patient to laceration or radiation."

But perhaps the best thing about the machine is that its price is so reasonable that it can be used in hospitals that could never afford costly apparatus. A GAI Tumor Detector costs about 110,000 yuan (US$13,200).

Patients who have experienced examinations by the GAI machine report it to be painless, except for a pins and needles sensation when the sensors touch their channel points.

Dr. Gai Guocai, however, admits that the machine has one weakness — it can only detect in which organ the tumor is located, but it cannot give the operator an indication in which part of the organ the tumor lies, nor its size. For this reason he advocates its use in conjunction with the CT scanner and X-ray.

In 1991, Gai and his son Gai Hua set up their own Beijing GAI Electronic Medical Apparatus Company Ltd. which has the capacity to produce 150 GAI machines each year. Gai machines are being used in dozens of hospitals across China.

FOR RELEVANT ILLUSTRATION, SEE Fig. 40.

CHAPTER 23

TEAMING UP WITH NATURE TO BEAUTIFY

Chinese women living in the Tang Dynasty (618-907AD) rouged their plump cheeks, plucked their eyebrows and painted hues of red on their lips. Centuries later, cosmetics were shelved for decades before China's reform and opening, being branded bourgeois. Acupuncturist Professor Tong Yujie has helped Chinese women make up for lost time and regain their reputation as beauties by world standards by re-formulating Chinese cosmetology, basing the art of beautification on the medical science of acupuncture, breathing, massage, food therapy and entirely natural cosmetics which combine to form the foundation for a beautifying lifestyle.

To many Chinese, the art of making up with cosmetics is a novel concept introduced from the West as recently as the early 1980s. Little do they know that China boasts the world's earliest records of applying natural medicines for beautification, dating back more than 2,000 years.

The Herbal Classic of Shen Nong, one of the earliest extant monographs on materia medica in the world, which dates back to the Qin (221-207BC) and Han (206BC-220AD) dynasties, lists over 20 kinds of "superior and medium (grade)" medicinal herbs as having cosmetic effects.

"For instance," Dr. Tong Yujie says, "the author of the ancient medical book recorded that Jade Bamboo, or fragrant solomonseal rhizome (*Rhizoma Polygonati Odorati*), can eliminate black spots on the face and beautify the complexion, while the dahurian angelica root (*Radix Angelicae Dahuricae*) is beneficial to human skin and can be made into facial cream."

Among the more than 1,892 medicinal substances noted in the *Compendium of Materia Medica*, authored by Li Shizhen (1518-1593) of the Ming Dynasty, 168 were specified as being effective against skin aging and for nursing damaged skin.

A graduate of the Harbin Medical College in northeast China's Heilongjiang Province and a Chinese medicine practitioner since the early 1950s, Tong is noted for his unique approach to cosmetology based on the theory and practice of traditional Chinese medicine. He is a guest professor lecturing in Chinese Medicine Cosmetology at the Beijing Union Medical College and has trained more than 1,500 students. Many of them have started their own beauty parlors based on Tong's teaching.

Change in Direction

But the professor is actually a late comer in the beauticians' world, despite his achievements in developing Chinese Medicine Cosmetology. In fact he confesses that he did not pay attention to cosmetology until 1983 when he participated in the Eighth World Acupuncture Conference in Bulgaria. He was attending the conference as an established acupuncturist and inventor of musical sound-wave acupuncture.

"Aside from the seminars and discussions, I was struck to see that nearly all the foreign female participants used make-up to enhance their natural beauty," Tong recalls. But none of the three Chinese women participants used any cosmetics. And when they were tempted to buy some, none of them knew how to apply them correctly.

It was understandable. A whole generation of Chinese had become alien to the concept of cosmetology due to the numerous political campaigns in the past decades, and above all, the Cultural Revolution (1966-76), when the use of any make-up was condemned as "bourgeois" and unacceptable in a proletarian country.

"My colleagues finally found an overseas Chinese in Bulgaria to teach them how to make up," he says. From her, Tong learned that there were lots of training courses around the world. Impressed, he was determined to master cosmetology.

"People in other countries view beauty products just as essential to life as food, clothing, housing and transportation," he observes. "But in China, women and men who are otherwise physically attractive might be disfigured by freckles, acnes, nevi, or warts. It's a pity."

Tong attended two cosmetology courses run by Hong Kong beauticians in 1985 and 1986, and was among the eldest but most eager students. He quickly realized that his expertise in traditional Chinese medicine could be put to use in cosmetology.

A Natural Way

"Conventional cosmetology usually uses cosmetics made from synthetic chemicals, and often deals with symptoms rather than root causes," Tong explains. "Where conventional cosmetology fails or is limited, systematic Chinese Medicine Cosmetology will search for the root cause and prescribe a fundamental cure."

He also notices the side effects of synthetic chemicals, saying that Chinese Medicine Cosmetology, using natural substances, should be safe and effective.

Based upon the theory of traditional Chinese medicine, Tong prescribes cosmetology which is non-invasive. It has five components: Chinese herbal medicine, acupuncture, massage, *qigong* (a system of deep breathing exercises with mind concentration), and food therapy.

A walking advertisement for Tong's Chinese Medicine Cosmetology is his second wife, Guo Xiaoqing. With a clear complexion, beautiful bright eyes, and a slender figure, Guo looks as if she's in her mid-30s, rather than her early 50s.

The former photographer now operates a beauty parlor in a residential area of Jinsong in southeastern Beijing.

"From time to time, people come here, just to look around. When they realize that I am 52, they hardly believe their eyes. Often on that basis alone they decide to be one of my clients," says Guo, a mother of two.

But before she came to know Dr. Tong, then a divorcee, in April 1995, Guo says she had deep wrinkles around her eyes and lips, butterfly spots on the cheek and flat warts on the backs of her hands. "And I never really cared about my looks after my first husband died of cancer five years ago," she says.

While she fell in love with the professor in his 60s, Guo was also amazed at his cosmetology. "With his own cosmetics, he eliminated all those butterfly spots and wrinkles and flat warts on my face and hands in a matter of two months," she says. "All my colleagues were surprised to see that I had became so much younger looking."

She quit her photographer's job and became one of Tong's students. In the summer of 1995, Guo opened her own beauty parlor.

Make Up Formula

What rejuvenated Guo's appearance is a line of cosmetics called *Wu Jing Yi Bai* in Chinese — five kinds of essence plus one whitener. It has been developed by Dr. Tong based on his studies of ancient Chinese prescriptions and preparations handed down over the generations. The major ingredients include musk, earthworms, powder of dried sea snake and pollen.

"The cosmetics made from these components are 98 percent successful in removing freckles, moles and birthmarks, warts, acne and unwanted facial hair," says the professor.

One of the most difficult dermatological problems is the elimination of freckles and brown spots. Dr. Tong can handle them with his cosmetology. One beneficiary is Sun Hong, a 25-year-old office clerk. Her face used to be covered with freckles, and none of the many beauty parlors and hospitals she visited could solve her problem. She was introduced to Dr. Tong in 1986.

The professor gave her a three-step therapy, namely, employing *qigong* to warm-up her respiratory system; massaging to relax her muscles and tendons; and applying the medicines — the five essences plus whitener — to remove the actual skin blemishes.

"Three days after the treatment, I was amazed to find most of my blemishes had faded — some had even disappeared," Sun recalls.

Sun also became a student of Dr. Tong and opened her own beauty parlor in Harbin, her home town, in 1987. She is among several of Tong's patients-turned-students who are now successfully operating parlors of their own.

Face Mask

One of the special features in the professor's cosmetology is his medicinal face mask. Made in seven varieties from more than 30 well-known Chinese medicines, including ginseng, Chinese angelica and musk, the paste-like maskings have different uses including those for anti-wrinkling (red), getting rid of acne (yellow), and nursing and whitening the skin (purple).

"They are effective because the penetrating fragrance of the natural medicines can stimulate the patient's cranial nerve system and speed up blood circulation, which will help the skin's absorption of the needed nourishment so as to have a skin cleansing and beautifying effect," he says.

The systematic Chinese Medicine Cosmetology puts stress on an overall analysis of each patient's unique physical condition before giving a treatment, says the professor. "That's what traditional Chinese medicine has emphasized," he explains. "People's needs for cosmetology vary from individual to individual, and from season to season."

His cosmetology also makes full use of acupuncture skills. Based on his invention of an electronic acupuncture instrument, he designed another device, also electronic, for accelerating the skin's absorption of Chinese medicine.

Tong spends much of his time teaching with the aim of spreading his conception of systematic Chinese medicine applied to beautification. Having trained more than 1,500 Chinese students, he set up in 1995 the Yujie International Training Center of Chinese Medicine Cosmetology at Zhangzhou in southeast China's Fujian Province. The center's intake mainly comprises students from Taiwan and Southeast Asia.

His introductory and middle-level courses trace the development of cosmetology both domestically and internationally, discuss skin care and beautification, and teach human anatomy. Other courses focus on techniques such as facial massage, face lifts, tattooing, and acupuncture. The advanced courses teach *qigong*, eyebrow and eye-line care and lip lines, and the design and use of electronic devices in cosmetology.

Chinese Medicine Cosmetology is being accepted by more and more people. But Tong is far from content. "My dream is to build a cosmetology center which integrates cosmetology, bodybuilding, food therapy, entertainment and beautician-training under one roof," he says.

CHAPTER 24

BREATHING LIFE BACK INTO THE PARALYZED

The master is the medicine in qigong. He possesses excess vital or biological energy and can impart it on others to heal. Wan Sujian's qigong can make crippled people walk again. Researchers cannot explain in scientific terms why this is so. But from experiments Wan has conducted on crippled piglets, he has proved that the enigmatic treatment he administers has nothing to do with superstition nor the power of will.

Even for most Chinese, let alone foreigners, *qigong* is a mysterious thing. What exactly is it? An exercise? A belief? A philosophy? A phenomenon? Medicine, magic or trickery?

One thing is for sure, it is misunderstood by many. It's a topic of chitchat within families as sons ask mothers why they get up at the crack of dawn, go to the park and stand statue-like still under trees in local parks — just breathing and sometimes flapping their arms.

That is the key: breathing. For *qigong* translates as "a system of deep breathing exercises." But it's not a new-fangled health kick. *Qigong* was probably invented about 25 centuries ago by the philosopher Lao Zi who lived from 604-531BC.

Perhaps the reason why *qigong* is so mysterious is that it has many branches and applications. Masters use it for improving health in general, curing ailments or even foreseeing the future.

Zhang Tongshou speaks positively about *qigong* — about what it's done for him in the past, not what's going to happen in the future. "*Qigong* has given me hope after a terrible accident five years ago," says the 53-year-old Beijing resident.

The nightmare happened in October 1991 when he fell at work and broke his back (the tenth vertebra). Surgery saved his life, but it was a life in a wheelchair. Operations could not repair his severely damaged spinal cord and nerves.

Zhang had no option but accept his disability. He spent the days sitting at home watching television. That proved to be his fortune.

He saw a program featuring the *qigong* practices of Dr. Wan Sujian in which a man seemingly condemned to a wheelchair for life was helped to walk. Zhang set about finding that doctor at the Beijing Institution of Medical *Qigong*.

Recalling his high hopes, Zhang says he half-expected Dr. Wan to perform some kind of miracle. " After a year's treatment I realized that *qigong* wasn't quack magic. It's a combination of traditional and modern therapies, but it really does work, gradually." Zhang can now walk at a pace of one kilometer per hour. Slow, but a real gift for a man who thought he'd never walk again.

Master Qualities

The man who gave the gift was Wan Sujian, 44. His main tools are his hands, or more accurately his palms.

They look thicker than those of ordinary men. The center of the palms have acupoints termed *Laogong* from where *qigong* masters release their internal *qi*, or vital energy. "I regard *qi* as a kind of biological energy - it exists in everyone, weak or strong, and it's this force that determines the health and longevity of each one of us."

People with large amounts of *qi* can pass it on to others. This is one form of *qigong* treatment, and the kind that Wan himself practices. Once transmitted, it dredges the recipient's *jingluo*, or meridian system of channels and collaterals, along which vital energy circulates. Another method of *qigong* is self-administered — the practitioner teaches the patient techniques to enable self practice.

Wan says that the outgoing *qi* radiated by the practitioner enables the patient to gradually drive out distracting thoughts and relax. As the *qi* flows through the patient's channels, it improves the responsiveness of the nervous system, helping to heal in the process, and reinforcing one's ability to resist disease.

In the clinic Wan practices as follows. The patient lies on a bed, is suspended, sits or stands, depending on his condition. The *qigong* master stands about one meter away, often flanked by his students.

When the *qigong* master starts to release *qi*, he stretches his arms outward. Then he begins to move his hands slowly but forcefully to gather up energy and transmit it to the patient. Sometimes the master will circle the patient, but he never actually touches him.

Recipient's Feelings

How does a patient feel when subjected to *qigong*? Zhang Ze, a 61-year old, describes it thus: "Very quickly I felt a kind of vibrating warmth, a bit like electricity, moving through my body. I began to shake a little, then quiver quite a lot. I couldn't stop myself. I also felt as if I was under the influence of magnetism. Then, when the master withdrew his arms, all the feelings stopped. It was so powerful."

Zhang sought Wan's help after having her esophagus largely removed with cancer. This tube, between the throat and the stomach, was reduced to just half-a-centimeter in diameter. That meant she could only drink a small amount of milk for each meal. She kept on with *qigong* for two years and over that time her ability to eat has improved remarkably and she now feels much better.

Dr. Wan gives *qigong* treatment along with other forms of therapy including acupuncture, massage, acupoints drug-injections and digital acupoints pressure as well as electrotherapy and magnetic-therapy.

He says that *qigong* is not a cure-all but is very effective as part of a treatment package particularly in cases of paraplegia for which Wan rates his work as effective in more than 84 percent of cases.

Catastrophic Beginnings

Wan entered the medical world as a result of catastrophe. Back in 1976 he led a military rescue group in the relief of Tangshan, the city in Hebei Province struck by a devastating earthquake. The tremor killed 240,000 and injured 160,000 others. Most injures involved the crushing of limbs under fallen masonry, many of which resulted in paraplegia. From that dreadful day in 1976 Wan has faced the challenge of helping people walk again.

After instruction from *qigong* masters, Wan realized that he had the ability to generate powerful *qi* himself. He also realized that this method of treatment was particularly effective for unblocking the *jingluo* (meridian system of channels and collaterals) and thus repairing the damaged nerves of paraplegics. While understanding the traditional practice of *qigong*, Wan experimented in subjecting patients to heavier doses of it — simply by having other *qigong* practitioners work alongside him.

To this end, he decided to recruit, train and manage his own group of practitioners. He sought students from poor, remote areas where medical care was hardly sufficient. He also took patients' children as students.

They underwent long, hard training programs involving studies of both Chinese and Western medicine and then *qigong* itself. Students had to keep themselves physically fit. After eight years of such preparations, the first batch of students earned their right to be *qigong* masters.

Maintaining *Qigong* Ability

Wan stresses that a master's hard work never stops. To maintain their skills they must train, but not overwork. His doctors train twice a day, getting up at 5 a.m. to exercise outdoors, no matter what the weather or season. The same training is repeated at night.

This physical fitness regime surprises many people. They tend to think *qigong* is some kind of psychological treatment like hypnotism. Wan explains: "I think *qi* is a material in the form of a transmitted message. If the *qigong* master sends out the right *qi* it will be able to work on the right part of the patient's body and open up their clogged *jingluo*. But if the message is wrong it can seriously disturb the biological order of the patient."

Pig Experiments

To prove his theory, Wan did something no other Chinese *qigong* master had done before. He conducted some experiments on animals.

Eighteen pigs were divided into three groups: A, B and C. They were all four months old and were genetically similar: all had the same father, but different mothers. The animals had their spinal cords injured in the same way.

Group-A pigs were given immediate treatment. The frequency was thrice a day for the first week, then twice a day for the rest of the time until 89 days had passed.

Group-B pigs commenced treatment later, a week after injury. But as with Group-A pigs they were treated thrice a day, then twice a day. This continued for 84 days.

Group-C pigs received no treatment.

Seventeen pigs survived. The six in Group-A were all able to walk. Two of them could even jump and run. Five animals in Group-B could stand up, with one of them being able to run and jump. None of the pigs in Group-C could stand up.

The effectiveness of treatment in the experiment speaks for itself. Dr. Wan says: "It's a pity that we can't explain exactly why *qigong* heals. But the pig test shows *qigong* has nothing to do with psychological suggestion or superstition."

Wan has developed different methods of *qigong* to treat paraplegia, cerebral thrombosis, semi-paralysis, traumatic ailments, infantile cerebral palsy, high blood pressure, and diseases of the central nervous system.

In recognition of these effective forms of *qigong*, Wan has won many accolades from home and abroad. He is regarded as one of the most influential *qigong* masters in the world and he co-founded the Beijing Institution of Medical *Qigong*. It is both a hospital and a school for the training and study of future masters.

Many of Wan's admirers are foreigners, proving they are undeterred by the mysteries of Chinese culture and its *qigong*. Irv Givot, a 51-year-old chiropractic doctor from Oregon in the United States, says: "It's true that we don't fully understand why *qigong* works, but when men first discovered that radio waves could carry sound they didn't understand that either."

Givot first came to Beijing to study under Wan in 1993 and, pleased with the results of taking his newly-acquired skills back to the U.S., he has returned to China several times since to learn more knowledge and skills.

Foreign Master

A most remarkable foreign *qigong* success story involves Dr. Richard Mayfield. He received the shocking news that his niece was comatosed and being kept alive by machine in a Wisconsin hospital. Mayfield

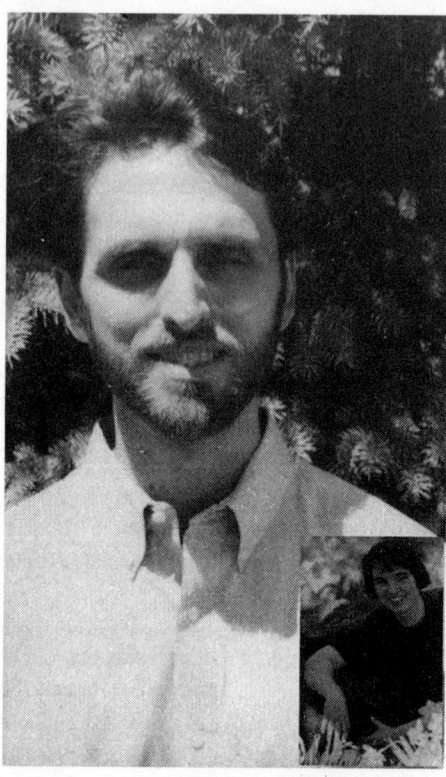

Dr. Richard Mayfield, who performed life-saving *qigong* on his comatosed niece in May, 1994.

Dr. Mayfield's niece, Leah Brisky, who recovered from the brink of death after receiving *qigong*.

immediately boarded an airplane in Minneapolis, practicing the techniques he'd learned from Wan during the flight. As soon as he got to his niece's bedside he started to release *qi*.

"In ten minutes the monitor showed that her brain activity was resuming," says Mayfield, "and, after a rest, I treated her for a further 20 minutes — then she opened her eyes."

Within six weeks she was out of her coma, smiling and able to move. "Now she is completely healthy — she graduated from high school recently," says Mayfield.

Wan's prestige among *qigong* followers around the world has aided the development of this, the most mysterious branch of traditional Chinese medicine. Donations he has received have helped him build a new hospital which opened in September 1996. Located at the foot of the Western Hills in Beijing, it consists of a teaching center, research block and 20 well-equipped wards.

It is sure to be the base at which many more discoveries concerning the effectiveness of *qigong* will be made — and a place where disabled people will learn to walk again.

FOR RELEVANT ILLUSTRATIONS, SEE Figs. 41-44.

CHAPTER 25

THE WORLD OF THE MEDICINE KING

In remote Tibet, a vast region of southwest China described as the Roof of the World for its altitude, an incredibly unique form of medicine has developed. Steeped in astrology and superstition it may be, but it is also based on sound medical approaches which combine with the abstract and immeasurable to form a fascinating, and as case histories show, an effective way of staying healthy and enjoying longevity in one of the earth's most hostile places.

When Demong Yangzong Zholma, a 78-year-old Lhasa woman, collapsed from a cerebral hemorrhage, doctors from the Regional Hospital of Tibetan Medicine sank a long needle into her head at an acupuncture point. Days later she was back to normal health.

Most Westerners would call such treatment a miracle, or even doubt that it could be performed, let alone be effective. In the world of traditional Tibetan medicine, however, both the practice and result are quite normal.

Yet considering Tibet, the vast plateau and mountainous autonomous region of southwest China, has been isolated by time and geography for centuries, it is logical that native people there should have developed a different way of doing things. And that includes a different approach to medicine.

Surgical theory and practice of Tibetan medicine dates back 2,000 years. It was initially based and limited to instinctive knowledge of human anatomy, explains Cering Bazhub, vice-president of the Regional Hospital of Tibetan Medicine. Thereafter, it only advanced in practical terms as a result of treating the bloody wounds of warriors dismembered in tribal warfare. By necessity, doctors became skilled in traumatology.

Buddhism's arrival in the 7th century was a turning point in the development of Tibetan medicine. United by religion, warfare became less common, which to a certain extent arrested progress in surgical practice. In the latter half of the 8th century, *the Four Medical Codices* were compiled. They were the earliest attempts to theorize on then-current practices, and they present contemporary scholars with a snapshot of traumatology more than a thousand years ago. Soon after, medical knowledge was presented in picture form as *thangkas*. The urge to record medical knowledge at the time was greatly influenced by the practice of learning and writing imported by Buddhism, whose temple monks copied out and translated sutras brought form Nepal.

More than 1,000 years later, in the late 1890s, the prince regent of Tibet, Samje Gyaco, instructed a group of Tibetan doctors, including an accomplished artist by the name of Lozha Dainzim Norbu, to standardize Tibetan medical theories on the basis of the ancient codices since Tibetan medicine had branched into several schools.

The sites of great learning were rock terraces, venues for "sky burials". The funerary procedure involved the dismemberment of corpses by *domdens*, or body breakers. (Vultures then ate the flesh and, according to belief, flew away and carried the soul of the deceased to heaven).

By witnessing the work of the *domdens*, doctors realized that the heart's shape and orientation was contrary to previous belief. This and other visual revelations enabled Dainzim Norbu to draw a series of 79 medical charts. To this day the works remain central not only to the teaching of Tibetan medicine, but also its practice.

"In fact," says Jampa Tiley, a noted Tibetan medical scholar and honorary president of the Regional Hospital of Tibetan Medicine, "the very existence of the Tibetan people on the Roof of the World owes much to indigenous folk medicine."

Ancient Tibetans, living in one of the world's most hostile regions, have long relied on charms, amulets and common sense as well as nature in maintaining good health. As early as the 3rd century BC, they had acquired the knowledge that where there is poison, there is medicine. In practice, they were then using yak-butter to stop bleeding and Tibetan barley-broth to cleanse external wounds.

Traditional Chinese medicine helped in the growth of its counterpart in Tibet. In the 6th century, ancient Han-Chinese medicine and astrology were introduced to Tibet, and in 641 AD, when Princess Wencheng of the Tang Dynasty (618-907) was diplomatically married off to Songtsan Gambo, the chieftain of the Tubo Dynasty of Tibet, she took her own medicines with her: she was equipped to treat 404 diseases. Packed in her baggage were also a number of medical books and instruments.

This Han-Chinese influence can still be seen today in some Tibetan medical practices, such as observation, investigation and taking of the pulse. Some herbs listed in Tibetan medical books were borrowed from Han medicine and are known by almost the same names.

Nevertheless, Tibetan medicine is unique in theory, diagnosis and practice, including acupuncture.

A major difference is that Tibetan doctors believe that human diseases are directly related to astronomical changes. Therefore, a good Tibetan doctor should also be an astrologist: astrological charts can be seen in all Tibetan hospitals.

Basic Diagnostics

As in traditional Chinese medicine, taking the pulse and checking the tongue are the main diagnostic methods employed by Tibetan doctors. Special attention is also placed on urine diagnosis, a unique and effective method adopted by Tibetan medical practitioners.

They analyze the patient's first morning urine. The urine of a fevered patient, for instance, is deep yellow, has a nauseating stench and is clouded with impurities.

Doctors of Tibetan medicine insist on using tailor's chalk in drawing lines to locate acupoints, instead of relying on experience as doctors of Chinese medicine usually do. Such caution is traditional, and is advised in the 8th century medical work, *The Four Medical Codices*. The importance of this book in Tibetan medical history can be compared with *The Yellow Emperor's Internal Classic*, the earliest medical book in China dating from the Warring States Period (475-221BC).

With *The Four Medical Codices*, systematic theories began to take shape.

Tibetan medicine holds that the human body is composed of seven materials including chyle, blood, flesh, fat, bone, marrow and reproductive glands. These materials work together to produce vital energy, internal heat and mucus for the body's operation. A person can remain healthy only when "the wind" through the skeleton, bile in the blood, phlegm in the flesh, fat and fluids are kept in equilibrium.

To ensure this, the theory says, proper diet, good living habits and medical tonics are essential. Medical treatment is listed only as the last resort.

Medical Drawings

Tibetans began to study the growth of the human body in the 7th century. Pictorially, medical *thangkas* (paintings on material) were produced to show their perception of human development from conception, through fetal development to birth. In the eyes of Tibetans, human embryology is a microcosm of evolution: one *thangka* depicts a fish, turtle and piglet appearing within a series of fetal stage-drawings and providing a fascinating parallel between human development and evolution. This theory existed 1,000 years earlier than that proposed by Charles Darwin.

Anatomical *thangkas* are used extensively to train today's doctors. To appreciate Tibetan medical theory in its widest sense, students study a tree of medicine whose roots, trunks, twigs and leaves are analogous to branches of medical practice ranging from embryology to pharmacology.

Good memory is a key quality for being a Tibetan doctor. They have to memorize ancient medical works and spend months in the wilds learning to identify medicinal herbs. Field trips usually last four weeks. A doctor is required to recognize more than 500 kinds of herbs. That number comprises one-sixth of the 3,000 types of Tibetan medical herbs known today.

"That is the first difficulty a student of Tibetan medicine has to overcome," Jampa Tiley says. "It's a necessary step to lay down a sound foundation, just like sharpening your axe before cutting firewood."

Traditionally, Tibetan medical knowledge and skills have been passed down from generation to generation as a family trade or by adopting apprentices. Today, medical schools and colleges have been opened in Tibet as a powerful additional means to carry forward the valuable heritage of Tibetan medicine.

Students of the Tibetan Medical College are chosen from high school graduates. A good educational background makes it easier for them to understand ancient medical classics.

Because of its effective cures and strict medical ethics, Tibetans tend to believe more in their folk medicine than in ready-made, boxed drugs.

"Our hospital is known among Lhasa's Tibetan residents as the City of the Medicine King," says Kunga Phuntsok, its vice-president. The Medicine King in Tibetan legends is an all-powerful medical wonder-worker.

Kunga's hospital, the regional hospital in Lhasa and the largest in the autonomous region, is where Demong Yangzong Zholma was cured seven years ago. The hospital's outpatient department treats 200,000 patients annually, nearly half of the total treated in all Chinese and Western clinics in the city.

The hospital receives the central government's financial support to the tune of more than three million yuan (US$ 385,000) per annum. With modern technology, the hospital's pharmaceutical factory manufactures 50,000 kilograms of Tibetan herbal drugs a year. Some 350 varieties are produced.

There are 12 other Tibetan-medicine hospitals in Tibet, and six outside.

Like traditional Chinese medicine in ancient times, modern science is also providing help wherever possible in the development of Tibetan medicine. The regional hospital, for instance, is equipped with all modern Western medical facilities available in the rest of China, except the CT scanning machine.

"We need scanners for further analysis and development of Tibetan medical theories," Jampa Tiley says. "For one thing, tradition cannot see the inside of a human body."

Jampa Tiley is optimistic about the future of Tibetan medicine. "With the help of modern facilities and techniques, traditional Tibetan medicine will have even better days ahead," he says.

FOR RELEVANT ILLUSTRATIONS, SEE Figs. 45-50.

CHAPTER 26

EVIDENCING THE EVOLUTION OF CHINESE MEDICINE

At the beginning of this century, a treasure house of Buddhist art was found in caves at Dunhuang in northwest China. Many precious relics found their way, usually illegally, abroad. Traveling to foreign museums more than 90 years later, Chinese researchers have discovered that many Dunhuang documents are revelations on early medical practices. Combined with studies of some of the cave murals, still in situ, they shed vivid light on the origins and early development of traditional Chinese medicine and its dissemination.

A study of manuscripts found in caves on the ancient Silk Road, and of the murals therein, has found many to be concerned with medical diagnoses and prescriptions, thus providing the contemporary medical profession and historians alike with an illustrated insight into the early development of traditional Chinese medicine.

The scrolls were found in the early 1900s, having been hidden behind walls in one of the caves at the Mogao Grottoes of Dunhuang, in northwest China's Gansu Province. The site was once a major religious center during the Sui and Tang dynasties (581-618, 618-907AD), the heyday of the Silk Road — an overland trade route linking China and Asia Minor via Central Asia — and it also served as an oasis where merchants rested, regenerated and worshipped before or after facing the hostilities of a desert crossing.

The discovery of the so-called "Library Cave" by Abbott Wang, containing a cache of thousands of manuscripts triggered instant international interest as a procession of archaeologist-adventurers converged on the remote oasis to obtain treasures for their own or their nations' collections. Hungarian-born Englishman Aurel Stein, and Frenchman Paul Pelliot took important relics away for their own collections which have since found their way into national collections in London, New Delhi and Paris respectively. Thus Chinese scholars have, to a large extent, been prevented from freely accessing the relics, particularly the more transportable ones such as scrolls.

In fact, systematic study of medical documents did not begin seriously until 1985 when Cong Chunyu, president of the Dunhuang Institute of Traditional Chinese Medicine, formed a six-person research team to visit museums in London and Paris. Cong describes the relics taken from Dunhuang's grottoes as "a treasure house" of traditional Chinese medicine, with almost all aspects of traditional medicine represented.

Lost Works

One achievement was the discovery of a considerable number of works, in manuscript form, detailing medical theories, certain herbal medicines and acupuncture, dating from the Sui and Tang dynasties. They are considered invaluable sources of information, filling gaps in the scarcely-existing medical literature remaining from that time.

Noteworthy was the finding of the only fragments of the long-lost *Commentary on The Herbal Classic of Shen Nong*, compiled by Tao Hongjing from the Southern Dynasties (420-589AD). The original seven-volume magnum opus, with more than 730 medicinal substances listed, was regarded as a guide for medical practitioners in ancient times.

The work is the earliest comprehensive commentary on *The Herbal Classic of Shen Nong*, the earliest extant monograph on materia medica in China. It is thought to have appeared as early as the Qin and Han dynasties (221-207BC, 206BC-220AD). Cong says the theory of using one drug to cure several kinds of illness, which was initiated by Tao and recorded in his works, can still guide today's clinical practitioners in their work.

Four scrolls were found to be early-stage developmental forms of China's first state-issued pharmacopoeia, *The Newly-Revised Materia Medica* which finally appeared in the Tang Dynasty. This appeared more than 800 years earlier than the noted *Nuremberg Pharmacopoeia* of 1542, thus highlighting the advanced nature of Chinese medicine at the time.

Experts learned from the document that it took less than eight years for the pharmacopoeia to spread from the then capital of China, in Chang'an (present-day Xi'an), to the border areas of the empire in the west.

Also found were fragments of *Dietetic Materia Medica*, a Tang monograph recording herbs which could be used as both foods and drugs. The original had been thought lost, though some text remained in the *Classified Materia Medica* and the *Ishinpo*, two monographs compiled by Japanese physician Yasurori Tanba (912-995AD).

Among the works were two important monographs on diagnosis and treatment based on the physio-pathological relationships between the five solid organs (heart, liver, spleen, lungs and kidneys) and the five sense organs (nose, eyes, lips, tongue and ears). They also dealt with the theory of five elements (metal, wood, water, fire and earth), one of the philosophies integrated with medical practice in ancient China and concerning the unity of the human body.

"These documents reflect an advanced level of medical science 1,000 years ago," says Prof. Cong. He notes the method of treating certain heart problems, such as angina pectoris, with niter-realgar powder "set beneath the tongue" or "swallowed with saliva to achieve a speedy effect."

Remarkably, this treatment was at least 1,000 years ahead of the appearance of its Western counterpart, which treats myocardial infarction and angina pectoris with glyceryl trinitrate set beneath the tongue or simply sniffed, Prof. Cong points out. The documents also included the earliest-known illustration of acupuncture.

Tibetan Medicine

Few Tibetan medical documents pre-Sui (before 581AD) and Tang dynasties were thought previously to be extant. But the team found that five scrolls taken by Stein and Pelliot, and lodged abroad, contained a wealth of information from this period. These documents were written before the eighth century, earlier than *The Four Medical*

Codices which are collectively regarded as the essential reference works for practitioners of traditional Tibetan medicine. They extensively listed prescriptions and methods of moxibustion.

Most noted among the findings are monographs detailing methods of moxibustion. They list six special ways of locating moxibustion positions from surface anatomy sense organs, examination of projecting bones or postures, and even by finger-pressing. Three illustrations of moxibustion points fill research gaps in Tibetan medical classics. Their 19 marked points prove that the study of moxibustion points was already well developed as early as the 7th and 8th centuries, says Prof. Cong.

"We have also found a theory about physio-pathological relationships between the five solid organs and the five sense organs, astonishingly similar to those of the traditional Chinese medicine," says Cong. "It clearly shows the common ground between Tibetan and Chinese medicines."

Prescriptions

Researchers were surprised to find as many as 1,024 prescriptions mentioned on different Buddhist scrolls. Most of the manuscripts are from the Sui and Tang dynasties and give a variety of prescriptions relating to surgical problems, gynecology, pediatrics, otorhinolaryngology (ear, nose and throat), ophthalmology, and dermatology. The experts were also fascinated by a considerable number of cosmetic preparations such as facial creams, hair tonics and shampoos. Most prescriptions epitomized, in one way or another, fundamental philosophies underpinning traditional Chinese medicine.

In the manuscripts concerning external treatments, many methods, such as fumigation and steaming, decoction-bathing, hot medicated compress application, gargling, inserting, and inducing (defecation by enema and suppository), are still valued by doctors as effective therapies today.

One prescription used by Daoists and Buddhists which particularly interested researchers was recorded on the back of a scripture. They found that the combination of the three ingredients mentioned, conidium fruit, schisandra fruit and polygala root, and recorded as being a sedative was in fact an aphrodisiac.

After two weeks of being given the medicine, white rats were found to have markedly developed utero-ovaries and testes. Further clinical experiments convinced researchers of the medicine's benefits in treating menstrual disorders, anemia and sterility, caused by ovulation dysfunction. "The textual study of the prescriptions is now being followed up with laboratory and clinical research," says Prof. Cong.

Imagery Medicine

Prof. Cong's team has identified 100 images showing aspects of medical and health work from the 45,000 square meters of Buddhist murals. These are still in situ, adorning the walls of the Mogao caves, many of which are now open to visitors.

Many paintings depict personal hygiene activities and attention to public sanitation. Activities such as teeth brushing, bathing and hair-cutting are common themes. "These pictures portray ordinary life on the ancient Silk Road," Cong says.

On the ceiling of Cave 302, dug in 584AD during the Sui Dynasty, two murals depict practitioners treating patients. A patient, naked, lies on a mat. His hands are held by two comforting, sympathetic relatives. Meanwhile the doctors make their examination. Elsewhere, a weak patient is raised into a sitting position while a practitioner prepares medicine. Such images are extremely rare records of ancient doctors at work.

The early morning mouth rinse appeared as early as the Warring States period (475-221BC). Basic teeth brushing developed in the Eastern Han period (25-220AD), with "brush-shaped willow twigs dipped in salt." Such a willow twig brush is depicted on a mural in Cave 159, which dates from the Tang Dynasty. In it, a monk can be seen applying salt to his teeth, while holding a cup with a brush.

Another mural shows a well enclosed by fences to guard against contamination, probably by domestic and farm animals. In Cave 296, dating from the Sui, a mural portrays a man toileting within a roofed structure — a lavatory.

A number of other murals show sporting activities including martial arts, *qigong* (a mind-concentrating cum deep-breathing exercise), and wrestling. "They reflect health consciousness in the lives of the ancients up to one thousand years ago," says Prof. Cong.

FOR RELEVANT ILLUSTRATIONS, SEE Figs. 51-53.

Appendix

WRITERS & CONTACT INFORMATION

A MEDICINE TO MOVE MOUNTAINS (Page 1-4)
(by *Chen Gengtao*)

Mr. Wang Changgen
Hangzhou Wang Changgen Special Clinic
for Liver, Gallbladder & Kidney Stones
317 Zhongshan Zhonglu
Hangzhou, 310001
Zhejiang Province
P.R. China
Tel (86-571) 7060234
Fax (86-571) 7062446

邮编: 310001
中国浙江省杭州市中山中路317号
杭州王长根肝胆肾结石专科门诊部
王长根　先生

FIGHTING POISON WITH POISON (Page 5-13)
(by *Yang Zheng*)

Mr. Hao Wenxue
Thrombus Hospital
Chinese Medical Sciences University
258 Bayi Road, Zhongshan District
Dalian, 116013
Liaoning Province
P.R. China
Tel (86-411) 2400315 / 2402131
Fax (86-411) 7611624

邮编: 116013
中国辽宁省大连市中山区八一路258号
中国医科大学血栓病医院
郝文学　先生

A HERBAL INJECTION TO CURE EPILEPSY (Page 14-19)
(by *Du Wenfeng* & *Zhao Qinghua*)

Mr. Zhao Zhanmin
Shanxi Pinglu Epilepsy & Encephalopathy Hospital
Pinglu County, 044300
Shanxi Province
P.R. China
Tel (86-359) 3522559 / 3522725

邮编: 044300
中国山西省平陆县中医癫痫脑病医院
赵占民　先生

FORGOTTEN POINTS OF ACUPUNCTURE (Page 20-24)
(by *Zhou Meiyue* & *Zhang Yu*)

Mr. Shi Huaitang
Apt #1, Entrance 3, Building 7
Western District, Jingang Neighborhood
Taiyuan, 030009
Shanxi Province
P.R. China
Tel (86-351) 3040481

邮编: 030009
中国山西省太原市金刚里西区7楼3单元1号
师怀堂　先生

TAKING THE PAIN OUT OF CONQUERING THE BIG C
(by *Pan Xiaoying*)　　　　　　　　　(Page 25-32)

Mr. Xie Tian
Zhejiang Kanglaite Pharmaceutical Co., Ltd.
#92-8 Longjing Road
Hangzhou, 310013
Zhejiang Province
P.R. China
Tel (86-571) 7986666 Ext. 2221
Fax (86-571) 7961873

邮编: 310013
中国浙江省杭州市龙井路92-8号
浙江康莱特药业有限公司
谢恬　先生

A DEADLY WEED: MEDICINE IN MEDICAL HANDS
(by *Liu Gongwu* & *Zhang Qi*)　　　　(Page 33-37)

Mr. Jin Zhanghong
Zhejiang DND Pharmaceutical Co., Ltd.
Ru'ao Town
Xinchang, 312560
Zhejiang Province
P.R. China
Tel (86-575) 6060282
Telefax (86-575) 6060164

邮编: 312560
中国浙江省新昌儒岙镇
浙江得恩德制药有限公司(原新昌第二制药厂)
金彰红　先生

THE POINT OF HEAT (Page 38-43)
(by *Wang Zhenshan* & *Xie Jinjin*)

Mr. You Fushan
Fire Needle Special Clinic
Rm 311, Building 10
Residential Compound
Lanzhou Bearing Factory
Lanzhou, 730050
Gansu Province
P.R. China
Tel (86-931) 2331154

邮编: 730050
中国甘肃省兰州轴承厂家属楼10号楼311室
由福山　先生

PUTTING ANTS TO WORK ON ARTHRITIS (Page 44-48)
(by *Li Hui* & *Sun Can*)

Ms. Sun Xiaoli
Nanjing Jinling Ant
Research and Treatment Center
307 Zhongshan Beilu
Nanjing, 210003
Jiangsu Province
P.R. China
Tel (86-25) 3424213 / 3346177 Ext.7343
Fax (86-25) 3428023

邮编: 210003
中国江苏省南京市中山北路307号
南京金陵蚂蚁研究治疗中心
孙晓莉　女士

REMOVING SOURCES OF PAIN WITH THE
BLADE-TIPPED NEEDLE　　(Page 49-60)
(by *Miao Hong*)

Mr. Zhu Hanzhang
Great Wall Hospital
China Academy of
Traditional Chinese Medicine
15 Zhengfu Street
Changping County
Beijing, 102200
P.R. China
Tel (86-10) 69742694
Fax (86-10) 69741595

邮编: 102200
中国北京市昌平县政府街15号
中国中医研究院长城医院
朱汉章　先生

A PHARMACY IN A TINY BOTTLE (Page 61-67).
(by *Yang Jianxiang* & *Liang Shutang*)

Mr. Peng Lirong
Yunnan White Medicine Group Co., Ltd.
51 Xiba Road
Kunming, 650032
Yunnan Province
P.R. China
Tel (86-871) 4141224
Fax (86-871) 4141473

邮编: 650032
中国云南省昆明市西坝路51号
云南白药集团股份有限公司
彭礼蓉　先生

THREADS SOAKED IN MYSTERY (Page 68-73)
(by *Chen Ya*)

Mr. Huang Jinming
Institute of Zhuang Medicine
Guangxi College of Traditional Chinese Medicine
21 Mingxiu Donglu
Nanning, 530001
Guangxi Zhuang Autonomous Region
P.R. China
Tel (86-771) 3137564 / 3131277
Fax (86-771) 3135812

邮编: 530001
中国广西壮族自治区南宁市明秀东路21号
广西中医学院壮医药研究所
黄瑾明　先生

MAKING LIFE LIVEABLE WITH AIDS (Page 74-79)
(by *Yang Zheng*)

Mr. Lu Weibo
AIDS Research Department
China Academy of Traditional Chinese Medicine
18 Beixincang, Dongzhimennei
Beijing, 100700
P.R. China
Tel (86-10) 64014411 Ext. 263
Fax (86-10) 64013896

邮编: 100700
中国北京市东直门内北新仓18号
中国中医研究院艾滋病研究室
吕维柏　先生

EASING COLD TURKEY TRAUMAS (Page 80-86)
(by *Yang Jianxiang*)

Mr. Duan Wenlong
Kunming Public Security Bureau
525 Beijing Road
Kunming, 650031
Yunnan Province
P.R. China
Tel (86-871) 3163309
Fax (86-871) 3161021 Ext.2444

邮编: 650031
中国云南省昆明市北京路525号
昆明市公安局
段文龙　先生

A HAIR RAISER FOR WIG WEARERS (Page 87-92)
(by *Zhao Qinghua*)

Mr. Zhao Zhangguang
Beijing Zhangguang 101 Group Corp.
725 Jinsong Xikou, Chaoyang District
Beijing, 100021
P.R. China
Tel (86-10) 67718965 / 65158960
Fax (86-10) 65158943 / 67710968

邮编: 100021
中国北京市朝阳区劲松西口725号
北京章光101集团公司
赵章光　先生

SOUTH CHINA'S PHARMACEUTICAL INSTITUTION
(by *Li Hui* & *Liu Gongwu*)　　　　　(Page 93-98)

Mr. Tang Changhua
Hangzhou Hu Qing Yu Tang Pharmaceutical Factory
78-10 Hanghai Road
Hangzhou, 310016
Zhejiang Province
P.R. China
Tel (86-571) 6992277 Ext. 6315 / 6995152
Fax (86-571) 6993828

邮编: 310016
中国浙江省杭州市杭海路78-10号
杭州胡庆余堂制药厂
汤昌华　先生

A HERBAL SWIPE AT MALARIA (Page 99-104)
(by *Zhou Meiyue* & *Liang Shutang*)

Mr. Guo Hongcai
Kunming Pharmaceutical Corp. Ltd.
Kunming Jinding Science & Technology Park
Kunming, 650100
Yunnan Province
P.R. China
Tel (86-871) 8182312
Fax (86-871) 8181968

邮编: 650100
中国云南省昆明金鼎科技园
昆明制药股份有限公司
郭鸿才 先生

SCALP ACUPUNCTURE: THERAPY CLOSE TO THE
SITE OF STROKES   (Page 105-110)
(by *Wang Zhengzhong*, *Miao Hong* & *Yang Zheng*)

Mr. Chen Daoyi
Scalp Acupuncture Hospital of
Traditional Chinese Medicine
Wangjiang County, 246202
Anhui Province
P.R. China
Tel (86-556) 7171391 / 7171581

邮编: 246202
中国安徽省望江县中医头针医院
陈道翼 先生

ATTACKING THE PARASITIC CULPRIT OF ACNE
(by *Zhou Meiyue*) (Page 111-115)

Mr. Zhao Zhongzhou
Yunnan Zhongzhou Pharmaceutical Co., Ltd.
Bagongli, Compound of the Army Institute
Kunming, 650207
Yunnan Province
P.R. China
Telefax (86-871) 7181554

邮编: 650207
中国云南省昆明市八公里陆军学院内
云南中州制药有限公司
赵中州　先生

REMEDIES FROM FOREST AND FAMILY (Page 116-120)
(by *Zhang Mingyou* & *Liu Zifu*)

Mr. Liao Hongyou
Guizhou Chinese Herbal Medicine Hospital
27 Chengji Road
Guiyang, 550001
Guizhou Province
P.R. China
Tel (86-851) 6850378 / 6824957

邮编: 550001
中国贵州省贵阳市城基路27号
贵州中草医医院骨伤结石专科门诊部
廖洪友　先生

A BREAK FROM TRADITIONAL PATIENCE (Page 121-125)
(by *Chen Ya*)

Mr. Liu Haifeng
Beijing Sanhua Hi-Tech Company
A-24 Fengtai Beilu
Beijing, 100071
P.R. China
Tel (86-10) 63812211 Ext. 3342
Fax (86-10) 63817138 / 64268292

邮编：100071
中国北京丰台北路甲24号
北京三花高科技公司
柳海峰　先生

FOR THE HEALTH OF NEWBORN BABIES (Page 126-132)
(by *Zhou Meiyue*)

Mr. Li Zhu
China Maternity & Infant Health Center
Beijing Medical University
38 Xueyuan Road, Haidian District
Beijing, 100083
P.R. China
Tel (86-10) 62091761
Fax (86-10) 62091141

邮编：100083
中国北京市海淀区学院路38号
北京医科大学中国妇婴保健中心
李　竹　先生

DETECTING SIGNALS OF DISTRESS FROM TUMORS
(by *Chen Ya* & *Miao Hong*)   (Page 133-138)

Mr. Gai Hua
Beijing Gai's Medical Instrument Co., Ltd.
2-1, Building 3
57 Enjizhuang, Haidian District
Beijing, 100036
P.R. China
Telefax (86-10) 68124059

邮编: 100036
中国北京市海淀区恩济庄57号3号楼2单元1号
北京市盖氏医疗设备有限公司
盖 华　先生

TEAMING UP WITH NATURE TO BEAUTIFY (Page 139-144)
(by *Zhou Meiyue*)

Mr. Tong Yujie
Shengzhuang Household Chemicals Co., Ltd.
46 Fengsheng Hutong, Xicheng District
Beijing, 100032
P.R. China
Tel (86-10) 66158915
Fax (86-10) 66158917

邮编: 100032
中国北京市西城区丰盛胡同46号
北京盛妆家化有限公司
佟玉杰　先生

BREATHING LIFE BACK INTO THE PARALYSED
(by *Xu Nan*)   (Page 145-151)

Mr. Wan Sujian
Qigong Research and Treatment Institute
A-3 Shaojiapo, Shijingshan District
Beijing, 100041
P.R. China
Tel (86-10) 66871784 / 66871783
Fax (86-10) 68879254

邮编: 100041
中国北京市石景山区绍家坡甲3号气功研治所
万苏健　先生

THE WORLD OF THE MEDICINE KING (Page 152-156)
(by *Li Hui* & *Xiong Lei* / contributing: *Doje Zhamdui*)

Mr. Gundui Dagyi
Tibetan Medicine Hospital of
Tibet Autonomous Region
14 Niangre Road
Lhasa, 850000
Tibet Autonomous Region
P.R. China
Tel (86-891) 6323428 / 6322573

邮编: 850000
中国西藏自治区拉萨市娘热路14号
西藏自治区藏医院
根堆达吉　先生

EVIDENCING THE EVOLUTION OF CHINESE MEDICINE
(by *Zheng Chunhua* & *Feng Cheng*)   (Page 157-161)

Mr. Feng Jianxin
Gansu College of Traditional Chinese Medicine
35 Dingxi Donglu
Lanzhou, 730000
Gansu Province
P.R. China
Tel (86-931) 8619986 / 8619329

邮编: 730000
中国甘肃省兰州市定西东路35号
甘肃中医学院
封建新　先生

CHINA FEATURES

Ms. Miao Hong
Medical Writer
China Features
P.O. Box 522
Beijing, 100803
P.R. China
Tel (86-10) 63074079 / 63073669
Fax (86-10) 63074358
E-mail: features@public.bta.net.cn
http://www3.east.cn.net/others/chinamed

邮编: 100803
中国北京522信箱
中国特稿社
苗红　女士

图书在版编目(CIP)数据

中医奇葩:英文/中国特稿社著.
-北京:新世界出版社,1997.9
ISBN 7-80005-322-9

I.中··· II.新··· III.中医治疗法-普及读物
IV.R242

中国版本图书馆 CIP 数据核字(97)第 08763 号

责任编辑:白瑾
版面设计:李辉

中 医 奇 葩

中国特稿社 著

*

新世界出版社出版
(北京百万庄路 24 号)
北京外文印刷厂印刷
中国国际图书贸易总公司发行
(中国北京车公庄西路 35 号)
北京邮政信箱第 399 号 邮政编码 100044
1997 年(英文)第一版 1997 年北京第一次印刷
ISBN 7-80005-322-9
03500
14-E-2762P

Postscript

BEHIND THE BOOK

This book is a collective effort by a group of professional feature-article writers and editors at China Features (est. 1950), based in Beijing, working with a network of local contacts throughout China. Most involved have worked and studied overseas, and in the course of their research for **UNBELIEVABLE CURES & MEDICINES FROM CHINA** traveled the length and breadth of the country over a one-year period. Clocking up tens of thousands of kilometers on their investigative travels, they heard medical theories and facts from eminent practitioners in cities and respected folk doctors in far-flung provinces. Questioning by training, the journalists saw treatments in progress and visited current and former patients concerned.

UNBELIEVABLE CURES & MEDICINES FROM CHINA is the third book from the China Features team. They authored **PORTRAITS OF ORDINARY CHINESE** (Foreign Languages Press, Beijing, 1990) to give readers an insight into the daily lives of Chinese from all walks of life. The book was also translated into German and published as **100 UNTER 1 MILLIARDE** (Westdeutscher Verlag, Germany, 1990). This was followed by **CHINESE WOMEN PARADE** (Xinhua Publishing House, Beijing, 1995) which focused on women's issues.

China Features accepts commissions for features on any aspect of Chinese life and culture and has 1,000 recipient clients in 120 countries. Its illustrated features have appeared in **Science** (USA), **Selecta-Verlag** (Germany), **Journal of Ambulatory Care Marketing** (USA), **Archeologia** (France), **Arts of Asia** (Hong Kong) and **The Hollywood Reporter** (USA). Photographs by James Z. Huang of China Features are regularly used by SYGMA.

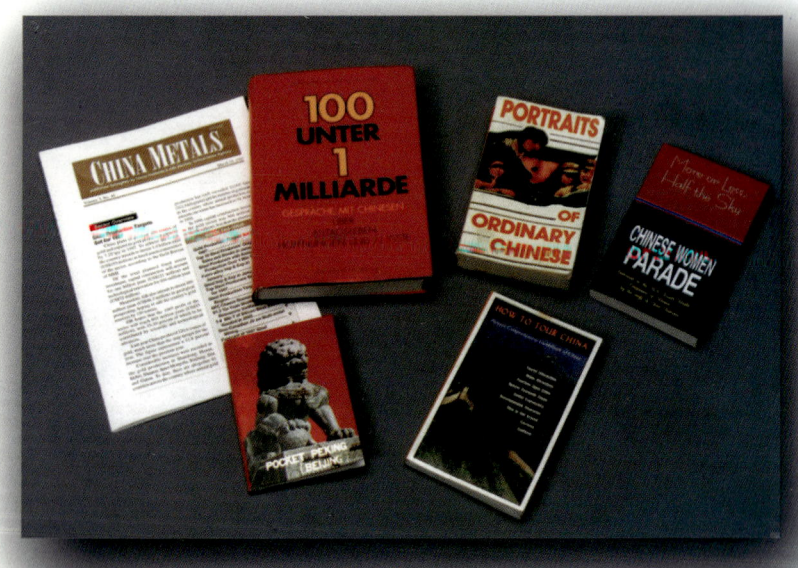

Books written by CF staff writers. CF also provides an information service, most notably CHINA METALS, a fortnightly publication which covers the latest developments in China's ferrous and non-ferrous metals industries.

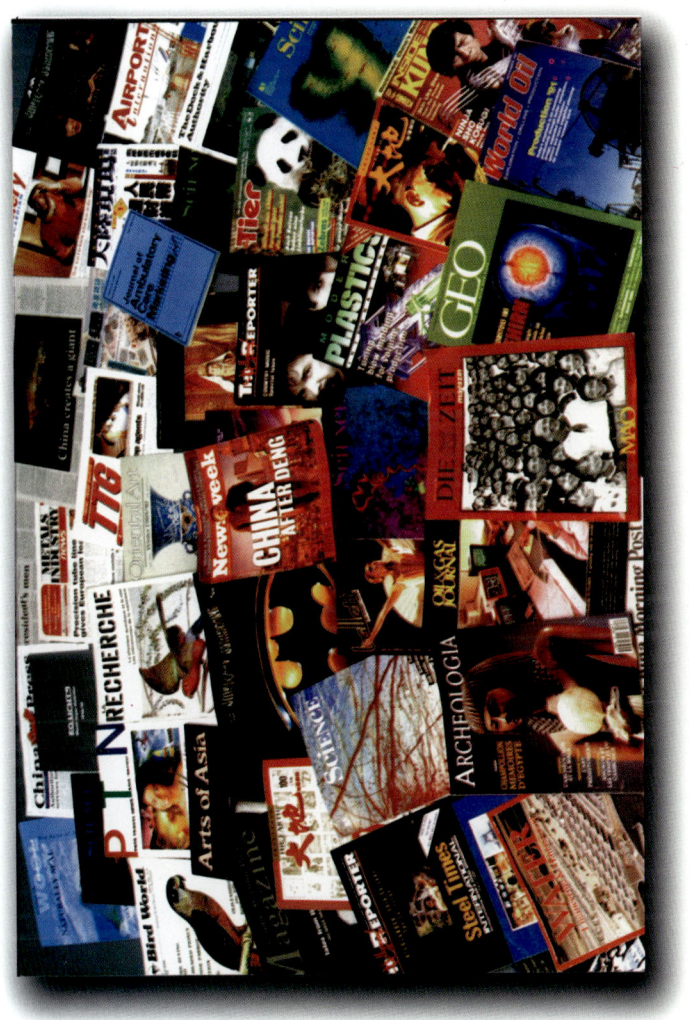

CF provides features and news photos for publications worldwide.

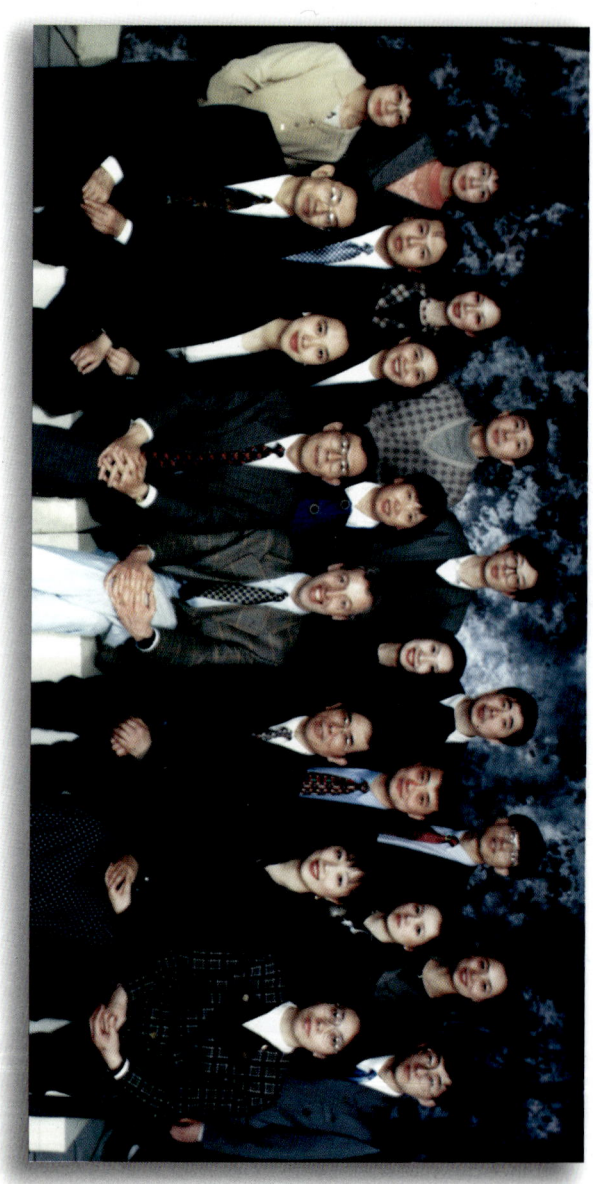

Staff writers and editors at China Features (CF). Front row from left: Zhao Qinghua, Pan Xiaoying, Chen Gengtao, William Lindesay, Li Zhurun, Yang Zheng and Chang Yanrui. Middle row from left: Ma Guihua, Wang Jue, Wang Hui, Xiong Lei, Miao Hong, Zhang Dan, Li Hui and Yang Jianxiang. Back row from left: Song Jingrong, Zhou Meiyue, Zhang Qi, Lu Xiaoming, Qu Jin, James Z. Huang and Bao Jiannu.

Extracts from the 12-volume *Plain Questions* which deals mainly with basic theories of medicine. These pages feature rearrangements and annotations by Wang Bing, a Tang-dynasty physician, who completed his editing in 762 AD after 12 years of work.

A 16th century edition of *The Yellow Emperor's Internal Classic*, China's oldest remaining medical work, written during the Warring States Period (475-221 BC). The 24-volume classic, of unknown authorship, consists of two parts: *Plain Questions* (Su Wen), and *Miraculous Pivot* (Ling Shu).

These wood-block printed books on stencil tissue paper, measuring 260mm × 174mm, were published during the Jiajing period (1522-1566) of the Ming Dynasty.

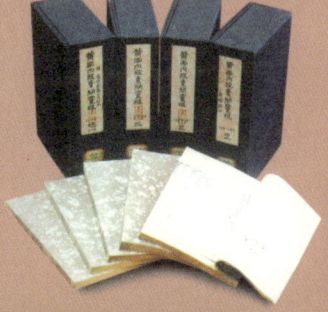

Photographs by courtesy of the library, China Academy of Traditional Chinese Medicine